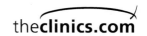

HEMATOLOGY/ ONCOLOGY CLINICS OF NORTH AMERICA

Integrative Medicine in Oncology

GUEST EDITORS
Moshe Frenkel, MD
and Lorenzo Cohen, PhD, MD

August 2008 • Volume 22 • Number 4

SAUNDERS

An Imprint of Elsevier, Inc.
PHILADELPHIA   LONDON   TORONTO   MONTREAL   SYDNEY   TOKYO

W.B. SAUNDERS COMPANY

A Division of Elsevier Inc.

1600 John F. Kennedy Boulevard • Suite 1800 • Philadelphia, Pennsylvania 19103-2899

http://www.theclinics.com

HEMATOLOGY/ONCOLOGY CLINICS
OF NORTH AMERICA
August 2008
Editor: Kerry Holland

Volume 22, Number 4
ISSN 0889-8588
ISBN 13: 978-1-4160-6307-0
ISBN 10: 1-4160-6307-2

Hematology/Oncology Clinics (ISSN 0889-8588) is published bimonthly by Elsevier Inc., 360 Park Avenue South, New York, NY 10010-1710. Months of issue are February, April, June, August, October, and December. Business and Editorial Offices: 1600 John F. Kennedy Blvd., Suite 1800, Philadelphia, PA 19103-2899. Customer Service Office: 6277 Sea Harbor Drive, Orlando, FL 32887-4800. Periodicals postage paid at New York, NY and additional mailing offices. Subscription prices are $262.00 per year (US individuals), $392.00 per year (US institutions), $131.00 per year (US students), $297.00 per year (Canadian individuals), $470.00 per year (Canadian institutions), $166.00 per year (Canadian students), $332.00 per year (international individuals), $470.00 per year (international institutions), $166.00 per year (international students). International air speed delivery is included in all *Clinics* subscription prices. All prices are subject to change without notice. **POSTMASTER:** Send address changes to *Hematology/Oncology Clinics of North America*, Elsevier Periodicals Customer Service, 6277 Sea Harbor Drive, Orlando, FL 32887-4800. Customer Service: 1-800-654-2452 (US). From outside the United States, call 1-407-563-6020. Fax: 1-407-363-9661. E-mail: JournalsCustomerService-usa@elsevier.com.

Reprints. For copies of 100 or more of articles in this publication, please contact the Commercial Reprints Department, Elsevier Inc., 360 Park Avenue South, New York, New York, 10010-1710; Tel.: 212-633-3813, Fax: 212-462-1935, and E-mail: reprints@elsevier.com.

Hematology/Oncology Clinics of North America is covered in *MEDLINE/PubMed (Index Medicus)*, *EMBASE/Excerpta Medica*, and *BIOSIS*.

Printed in the United States of America.

ELSEVIER
SAUNDERS

HEMATOLOGY/ONCOLOGY CLINICS
OF NORTH AMERICA

Integrative Medicine in Oncology

GUEST EDITORS

MOSHE FRENKEL, MD, Associate Professor of Integrative Medicine, and Medical Director, Integrative Medicine Program, The University of Texas M.D. Anderson Cancer Center, Houston, Texas

LORENZO COHEN, PhD, MD, Professor and Director, Integrative Medicine Program, The University of Texas M.D. Anderson Cancer Center, Houston, Texas

CONTRIBUTORS

MARC IAN BARASCH, Boulder, Colorado

ERAN BEN-ARYE, MD, Complementary and Traditional Medicine Unit, Department of Family Medicine, Faculty of Medicine, Technion-Israel Institute of Technology; Clalit Health Services, Haifa, Israel

KATE BODDY, MA, Information Officer, Complementary Medicine, Peninsula Medical School, Universities of Exeter and Plymouth, Exeter, United Kingdom

BARRIE CASSILETH, MS, PhD, Laurance S. Rockefeller Chair in Integrative Medicine and Chief, Integrative Medicine Service, Memorial Sloan-Kettering Cancer Center, New York, New York

LORENZO COHEN, PhD, MD, Professor and Director, Integrative Medicine Program, The University of Texas M.D. Anderson Cancer Center, Houston, Texas

ELIZABETH DEAN-CLOWER, MD, MPH, Public Health Physician in Integrative Oncology, Harvard Medical School; Leonard P. Zakim Center for Integrative Therapies, Dana-Farber Cancer Institute, Boston, Massachusetts

ANNE DOHERTY-GILMAN, MPH, Program Manager, Leonard P. Zakim Center for Integrative Therapies, Dana-Farber Cancer Institute, Massachusetts

EDZARD ERNST, MD, PhD, FRCP, FRCPEd, Professor of Complementary Medicine, Peninsula Medical School, Universities of Exeter and Plymouth, Exeter, United Kingdom

NICOLE FLORY, PhD, Postdoctoral Fellow and Associate Director, Nonpharmacologic Analgesia Program, Department of Radiology, Beth Israel Deaconess Medical Center, Harvard Medical School, Boston, Massachusetts

MOSHE FRENKEL, MD, Associate Professor of Integrative Medicine, and Medical Director, Integrative Medicine Program, The University of Texas M.D. Anderson Cancer Center, Houston, Texas

OFRA GOLAN, LLD, Department for Complementary/Integrative Medicine, Law, and Ethics, International Center for Health, Law, and Ethics, Haifa University, Haifa; Unit for Genetic Policy and Bioethics, Gertner Institute for Epidemiology and Health Policy Research, Tel Hashomer, Israel

JAMES S. GORDON, MD, Founder and Director, The Center for Mind-Body Medicine; Clinical Professor, Department of Psychiatry; and Clinical Professor, Department of Family Medicine, Georgetown University School of Medicine, Georgetown University Medical Center; Creator, CancerGuides® Training Program, Washington, District of Columbia

JYOTHIRMAI GUBILI, MS, Assistant Editor, Integrative Medicine Service, Memorial Sloan-Kettering Cancer Center, New York, New York

MARY L. HARDY, MD, Medical Director, Simms/Mann–UCLA Center for Integrative Oncology, University of California at Los Angeles, Los Angeles, California

ELVIRA LANG, MD, FSIR, FSCEH, Associate Professor of Radiology and Director, Nonpharmacolgic Analgesia Program, Department of Radiology, Beth Israel Deaconess Medical Center, Harvard Medical School, Boston, Massachusetts

ANNE LEIS, PhD, Dr. Louis Schulman Cancer Research Professor and Associate Professor, Department of Community Health and Epidemiology, University of Saskatchewan, Saskatoon, Saskatchewan, Canada

WEIDONG LU, MB, MPH, Lic Ac, Staff Acupuncturist, Harvard Medical School; Leonard P. Zakim Center for Integrative Therapies, Dana-Farber Cancer Institute, Boston, Massachusetts

CYNTHIA D. MYERS, PhD, LMT, NCTMB, Assistant Professor and Director, Integrative Medicine, Health Outcomes and Behavior Program, Moffitt Cancer Center, Tampa, Florida

RACHEL NAOMI REMEN, MD, Institute for the Study of Health and Illness at Commonweal, Bolinas; Professor of Clinical Medicine, Department of Family and Community Medicine, University of California, San Francisco, San Francisco, California

DAVID S. ROSENTHAL, MD, Professor of Medicine, Harvard Medical School; Medical Director, Leonard P. Zakim Center for Integrative Therapies, Dana-Farber Cancer Institute; Henry K. Oliver Professor of Hygiene, Harvard University, Boston, Massachusetts

ELAD SCHIFF, MD, Department of Internal Medicine, Bnai-Zion Hospital; Department for Complementary/Integrative Medicine, Law, and Ethics, International Center for Health, Law, and Ethics, Haifa University, Haifa, Israel

BRENT J. SMALL, PhD, Associate Professor, Health Outcomes and Behavior Program, Moffitt Cancer Center, Tampa, Florida

MARJA J. VERHOEF, PhD, Professor and Canada Research Chair in Complementary Medicine, Department of Community Health Sciences, University of Calgary, Calgary, Alberta, Canada

TRACY WALTON, LMT, MS, Training and Consultation: Caring for Clients with Cancer, Cambridge, Massachusetts

K. SIMON YEUNG, PharmD, LAc, Research Pharmacist, Integrative Medicine Service, Memorial Sloan-Kettering Cancer Center, New York, New York

HEMATOLOGY/ONCOLOGY CLINICS
OF NORTH AMERICA

Integrative Medicine in Oncology

CONTENTS   VOLUME 22 • NUMBER 4 • AUGUST 2008

Conventional wisdom generally recommends complete avoidance of all dietary supplements, especially during chemotherapy and radiation. This interdiction persists, in spite of high rates of dietary supplement use by patients throughout all phases of cancer care, and can result in patients' perceptions of physicians as negative, thus leading to widespread nondisclosure of use. A review of the clinical literature shows that some evidence for harm does exist; however, data also exist that show benefit from using certain well-qualified supplements. Physicians should increase their knowledge base about dietary supplement use in cancer and consider all of the data when advising patients. Strategies that are patient-centered and reflect the complete array of available evidence lead to more nuanced messages about dietary supplement use in cancer. This should encourage greater disclosure of use by patients and ultimately increase safety and efficacy for patients choosing to use dietary supplements during cancer care.

Health care professionals, patients, and care givers require access to good quality, reliable information about integrative oncology. Despite the vast resources available, it can be difficult to find objective, evidence-based information. This article provides an overview of reliable integrative oncology information from various resources. Selection methods are detailed and evaluation performed using a validated instrument. Resources that met the selection criteria and produced high evaluation scores are reviewed in detail. Resources include research databases, clinical databases, online information systems, and print media.

address the challenges faced by biomedical research methodology when applied to cancer care. In addition, they identify new research directions to meet these challenges. These include qualitative research, mixed methods research, and approaches based on systems thinking.

Mind-body medicine, grounded in a respectful, therapeutic partnership, should be a central element in the care of every person diagnosed with cancer. This article reviews some of the physiologic foundations of mind-body medicine, the introduction of mind-body approaches to cancer care in the 1970s, the specific mind-body approaches that have been used, and the evidence that supports their use. The importance of group support for enhancing the effectiveness of these approaches is discussed. Guidelines are offered for integrating mind-body approaches and perspectives in the care of people who have cancer.

Novel advances in biotechnology and medical imaging techniques have enabled an evolution toward earlier diagnosis and treatment by way of "minimally invasive" surgical techniques performed on the conscious patient without the use of general anesthesia. Although the risks of diagnostic and therapeutic interventions have been reduced with these approaches, patients still face many physical and psychologic challenges. Several randomized controlled trials have shown that hypnotic techniques are effective in reducing pain, anxiety, and other symptoms; in reducing procedure time; and in stabilizing vital signs. The benefits of adjunctive hypnotic treatments come at no additional cost. Patients, health care providers, hospitals, and insurance companies are advised to take advantage of hypnotic techniques.

This article provides a model of integrating complementary and integrative medicine into cancer care in a comprehensive conventional cancer center. This model requires a patient-centered approach with attention to patients' concerns and enhanced communication skills. A discussion of patients' psycho-social-spiritual perspectives is a crucial component in this approach. In addition, complementary and integrative medicine practitioners and conventional practitioners' involvement and cooperation in developing this integration process are essential. This process requires tremendous team effort, institutional culture change, trust and open communication between all members of the health care team, and support from institutional leaders.

Integrative oncology relates to an emerging dialog between complementary and alternative medicine (CAM) scholars, oncologists, family practitioners, and other health care providers who envision an extended and holistic patient-centered approach to oncology care. The multiple commitments of integrative oncology to a medical humanistic approach and to a strong evidence-based foundation may impose considerable ethical concerns and dilemmas. The authors use narrative ethics to present a case study that exemplifies the ethical challenges confronting physicians and health care providers who wish to provide an integrative approach for their patients. An ethical analysis of the narrative is provided to help clarify the ethical issues and conflicts within it. Finally, a framework that may transform ethical constraints to a communication tool is proposed.

Mind-body therapies are often portrayed in the literature as self-palliative, adjunctive, and complementary, but rarely as contributive to cure. Many physicians continue to view them as acceptable indulgences so long as they are harmless and the patient remains fully compliant with a standard treatment regimen. The possibility that such modalities might help drive the healing process itself is infrequently acknowledged. This article addresses the topic of such therapies, examining remarkable recoveries in cancer, and suggesting the need for a "Remarkable Recovery Registry" to expand the literature on these cases. The author discusses the importance of complementary alternative medicine, and emotional and pyschologic support in the treatment regimen, and the need for health care providers and patients to work together to provide the best emotional environment for the healing process.

Integrative medicine has been defined in several ways. For some it is a discipline that combines such approaches to the resolution of disease as acupuncture and homeopathy, meditation and imagery with more familiar and accepted health practices, such as surgery, pediatrics, and oncology. For others it is about cultivating awareness and sensitivity beyond symptoms to the mental, emotional, and spiritual needs of the patient. But, integrative medicine is more than the weaving together of techniques, or understanding the intimate interaction of the mental, emotional, and spiritual dimensions of human experience. It is about rethinking the task of medicine and the infrastructure of relationships and beliefs that have limited its power to serve all people.

Hematol Oncol Clin N Am 22 (2008) xi

HEMATOLOGY/ONCOLOGY CLINICS
OF NORTH AMERICA

ERRATUM

Relapsed and Refractory Hodgkin's Lymphoma: New Avenues?

George P. Canellos, MD

Harvard Medical School, Dana-Farber Cancer Institute, 44 Binney Street, Boston, MA 02115, USA

In the above article, which published in the October 2007 issue of the *Hematology/Oncology Clinics of North America* (volume 21, issue 5), please note that further clarification is needed in Table 2 on page 933. The cisplatin dose is 75 mg/m^2 on day 1 only, not day 1 and day 8 as appears in the table.

0889-8588/08/$ – see front matter
doi:10.1016/j.hoc.2008.06.002

HEMATOLOGY/ONCOLOGY CLINICS
OF NORTH AMERICA

HEMATOLOGY/ONCOLOGY CLINICS
OF NORTH AMERICA

Preface

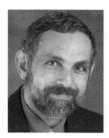 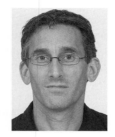

Moshe Frenkel, MD
Lorenzo Cohen, PhD, MD

Guest Editors

C omplementary and alternative medicine has been defined by the National Center for Complementary and Alternative Medicine and major U.S. surveys as "...diverse medical and healthcare systems, practices, and products that are not presently considered to be part of conventional medicine" [1]. Complementary therapies include mind-body approaches (such as meditation, guided imagery, music, art, and other behavioral techniques), energy-based therapies (such as yoga, tai chi, qigong, Reiki, and healing touch); body-manipulative approaches (such as chiropractic and massage), alternative medical approaches (such as traditional Chinese medicine, homeopathy, and Ayurveda), and biologic based approaches (such as those centered on nutrition, herbs, plants, and animal, mineral, or other products). Several different specialty health care providers offer complementary and alternative medicine therapies, which may include physicians, nurses, physical therapists, psychiatrists, psychologists, chiropractors, massage therapists, and naturopaths who are operating within the guidelines of their licenses or accrediting organizations.

The terms *alternative*, *complementary*, and *conventional* focus on treatment modalities. In the last few years, the term *integrative medicine* or complementary and integrative medicine (CIM) has become more prevalent in medical academia. Integrative medicine is more about a philosophy of medical practice. The Consortium of Academic Health Centers for Integrative Medicine has defined this term as "the practice of medicine that reaffirms the importance of the relationship between practitioner and patient, focuses on the whole person, is informed by evidence, and makes use of all appropriate therapeutic approaches, healthcare professionals and disciplines to achieve optimal health and healing" [2].

0889-8588/08/$ – see front matter
doi:10.1016/j.hoc.2008.06.001

There is a tremendous interest and use of CIM nationwide, and among patients and families touched by cancer, the use is higher than in the general population. In some studies, over 30% of patients and up to 83% of patients who have cancer use CIM [3,4], and most studies estimate that at least 50% of patients use CIM at some point in their journey.

In most cases, people who use CIM are not disappointed or dissatisfied with conventional medicine, but they want to do everything possible to regain health and to improve their quality of life [5–10]. Patients use CIM to reduce side effects and organ toxicity, to improve quality of life, to protect and stimulate immunity, or to prevent further cancers or recurrences.

The extensive use of CIM is a challenge to health care professionals who typically have limited knowledge of this "new" area and who have limited time to reeducate themselves. At the same time, patients can become frustrated and are not understood if they cannot discuss CIM with their physician. This bilateral frustration can result in a communication gap, which damages the patient-physician interaction. The most common reason patients give for not bringing up an interest in or use of CIM is that it just never came up in the discussion; that is, no one asked them, and they did not think it was important. Patients may fear that the topic will be received with indifference or will be dismissed without discussion [11,12], and health care professionals may fear not knowing how to respond to questions or may fear initiating a time-consuming discussion. As a result, it is estimated that 38% to 60% of patients who have cancer are taking complementary medicines without informing any member of their health care team [13,14]. This lack of discussion is of grave concern, especially for ingestible substances.

Physicians' failure to communicate effectively with patients about CIM may result in a loss of trust within the therapeutic relationship. In the absence of physician guidance, patients may choose harmful, useless, ineffective, and costly complementary therapies, when effective CIM therapies may exist. The erosion in trust caused by the lack of communication also can lead to decreased compliance with conventional medicine and certainly refusal to comply with the physician's advice about CIM use. Poor communication also may lead to a patient's diminished autonomy and sense of control over their treatment, thereby interfering with the self-healing response [11,12].

While scientific and evidence-based thinking is fundamental to contemporary medical practice, patients often do not reason in this way. A physician's failure to recognize this interferes with their ability to address the unspoken needs of patients. Psychological, social, and spiritual dimensions of care may be ignored if physicians cannot adapt to the individual needs of the patient or do not provide care with sensitivity. When physicians are faced with unfamiliar information about CIM therapies, they may feel "de-skilled" by being forced outside their medical specialty. This discomfort can lead to defensiveness and a breakdown in communication with the patient. In contrast, the physician who is receptive to patient inquiries and aware of subtle, nonverbal messages can create an environment in which a patient feels protected and can openly discuss potential CIM choices [11,15].

As CIM practice in cancer care grows and patients are exposed to non-biomedical therapeutic models, oncology clinicians increasingly are faced with patients requesting (or expecting) discussion about such issues in medical consultations. The increased use of CIM in cancer care is raising important challenges and questions about the oncology clinician's knowledge of and attitude toward CIM, the approaches to CIM in oncology consultations, and the implications for patient care. Certainly, existing research suggests that the vast majority of cancer patients desire communication with their doctors about CIM [16], and there is general agreement within the oncology community that oncologists must be aware of CIM use and be able to guide their use of all therapeutic approaches in order to provide effective patient care [17,18]. It is the health care professional's responsibility to ask patients about use of complementary medicines. Optimally, the discussion should take place before the patient starts using a complementary treatment. A number of strategies can be used to increase the chance of a worthwhile dialogue. Underlying these specific strategies should be an open attitude combined with a willingness to review evidence-based references and consult with other health care professionals [19].

Although applying the concept of integrative medicine to cancer care is still in its infancy, a number of comprehensive cancer centers in the United States are trying to put this concept into practice under the term "integrative oncology". As a result of this growing interest in integrative medicine in cancer care, the Society for Integrative Oncology (SIO) was established in 2003. In the SIO mission statement, the society describes itself as being dedicated to studying and facilitating cancer treatment and recovery through the use of integrated complementary therapeutic options, including natural and botanical products, nutrition, acupuncture, massage, mind-body therapies, and other complementary modalities [20]. The Journal of the Society for Integrative Oncology is a peer reviewed, Medline indexed journal dedicated to publishing original research and educating within the filed of integrative oncology.

In this issue of the *Hematolgy/Oncology Clinics of North America*, we have assembled a diverse set of articles from world renowned experts in integrative medicine and integrative oncology. When reading this issue you will be exposed to the evidence, theories, research challenges, and philosophy of integrative oncology.

Dr. Hardy from the University of California, Los Angeles discusses the most commonly used CIM in cancer care: nutritional supplements. The controversy surrounding this topic in cancer care is clarified and reviewed. Dr. Hardy provides a very comprehensive review of possible beneficial supplements that can be considered in integrative oncology. However, as you review her comments, you may wonder how get up-to-date and reliable information sources to provide advice and educate patients. Drs. Boddy and Ernst from the United Kingdom took on this challenge, and they review how to locate and use reliable information sources needed to provide appropriate integrative oncology care. They provide a comprehensive review of how to search for those resources and bring practical examples and suggestions for current available Web sites.

Dr. Lu and his colleagues from the Dana Farber Cancer Institute review the use of acupuncture in cancer care. This therapy has been around for more than 3000 years and is a commonly used CIM practice. In cancer care, it has been used successfully to improve quality of life, sleep, appetite, pain, and nausea after chemotherapy. Dr. Lu further explores the issue of research and support for the use of acupuncture in cancer care.

Dr. Myers discusses the use of massage therapy in cancer care. Massage is another commonly used approach to improve quality of life in patients suffering from cancer. Massage can reduce anxiety and tension, a symptom experienced by most people who have cancer and other cancer-related symptoms.

The topic of researching integrative oncology practices is quite complex. Drs. Yeung, Gubili, and Cassileth from the Memorial Sloan-Kettering Cancer Center examine evidence-based research on herbal therapies and the complexities related to researching these agents, including selecting an appropriate study method and clinical trial design, navigating through regulatory obstacles, and obtaining funding. They emphasize how evidence-based botanical research can help validate traditional uses and facilitate new drug development.

Drs. Verhoef and Leis from Canada bring a unique outlook on the limitations of current research methodology used in cancer care. They emphasize that cancer care is a complex package of a wide range of interventions often complemented by self- and supportive-care. They review the challenges faced by biomedical research in cancer care and discuss new research directions to meet these challenges. They examine the value of qualitative research and whole systems research methods as possible research, which are especially relevant in the field of integrative oncology and conventional oncology when examining personalized medicine.

The mind-body connection is an extremely important topic being discussed in most integrative oncology practices, and Dr. Gordon provides a comprehensive review on this topic. He elaborates on the scientific evidence on stress and cancer and discusses the multiple options available for stress reduction. The mind-body connection is an important aspect of integrative oncology and is further emphasized in the recent Institute of Medicine report [21]. This comprehensive report states, "cancer care today often provides state-of-the-science biomedical treatment, but fails to address the psychological and social (psychosocial) problems associated with the illness. These problems – including... anxiety, depression or other emotional problems... – cause additional suffering, weaken adherence to prescribed treatments, and threaten patients' return to health" [21]. As Dr Gordon suggests, mind-body interventions appear to address many of the issues mentioned in the Institute of Medicine report.

Drs. Flory and Lang from Harvard University discuss the practicality of how mind-body interventions are successfully used in the diagnostic radiology domain and how effective those techniques are in reducing morbidity and cost to the health care system.

We present our experience in integrative oncology from The University of Texas M.D. Anderson Cancer Center. We describe how a program of integrative oncology can encompass the different aspects of integrative oncology and how they are integrated into a large comprehensive cancer center in a real life setting.

Drs. Ben-Arye, Schiff, and Golan from Israel provide a distinct dimension on integrative oncology and ethics. They review a case presentation and examine the multiple issues related to ethical dilemmas in using integrative medicine in cancer care, with practical important suggestions for future patient care.

Mr. Barasch provides a unique perspective on remarkable recoveries. He brings his perspective on exceptional patients who had an unusual and unexpected recovery from their illness. His views are based on his personal experience as a patient and as an author of a New York Times best seller book *Remarkable Recovery* [22].

In this issue of *Hematolgy/Oncology Clinics of North America*, we have tried to provide an overview of integrative oncology as a new evolving field in medicine. We approached integrative oncology in a bio-psychosocial-spiritual manner. We start with specific issues that relate to the "physical body" and evidence-based research and practice. This is followed by examination of the psyche and the social context in relationship to health and healing. We end with "the spirit", as noted in Dr. Remens' profound article, presenting stories that highlight the meaning of our practice. We see this issue as a stimulus and a base for further discussion and research, and we hope that it surprises you, at times touches your heart, and mostly inspires you.

Moshe Frenkel, MD
Lorenzo Cohen, PhD, MD
Integrative Medicine Program
The University of Texas
M.D. Anderson Cancer Center
1515 Holcombe Boulevard, Unit 145
Houston, TX 77030, USA

E-mail addresses: mfrenkel@mdanderson.org;
lcohen@mdanderson.org

References

[1] National Center for Complementary/Alternative Medicine of the National Institutes of Health. What is complementary and alternative medicine? Available at: http://nccam.nih.gov/health/whatiscam/. Accessed March 8, 2008.

[2] Consortium of Academic Health Centers for Integrative Medicine. Definition of integrative medicine. Available at: http://www.imconsortium.org/cahcim/about/home.html. Accessed June 12, 2008.

[3] Richardson MA, Sanders T, Palmer JL, et al. Complementary/alternative medicine use in a comprehensive cancer center and the implications for oncology. J Clin Oncol 2000;18(13):2505–14.

[4] Ernst E, Cassileth BR. The prevalence of complementary/alternative medicine in cancer: a systematic review. Cancer 1998;83(4):777–82.

[5] Crocetti E, Crotti N, Feltrin A, et al. The use of complementary therapies by breast cancer patients attending conventional treatment. Eur J Cancer 1998;34(3):324–8.

[6] Miller M, Boyer MJ, Butow PN, et al. The use of unproven methods of treatment by cancer patients. Frequency, expectations and cost. Support Care Cancer 1998;6(4):337–47.

[7] Wyatt GK, Friedman LL, Given CW, et al. Complementary therapy use among older cancer patients. Cancer Pract 1999;7(3):136–44.

[8] Morant R, Jungi WF, Koehli C, Senn HJ. [Why do cancer patients use alternative medicine?]. Schweiz Med Wochenschr 1991;121(27-28):1029–34.

[9] Kappauf H, Leykauf-Ammon D, Bruntsch U, et al. Use of and attitudes held towards unconventional medicine by patients in a department of internal medicine/oncology and haematology. Support Care Cancer 2000;8(4):314–22.

[10] Oneschuk D, Fennell L, Hanson J, Bruera E. The use of complementary medications by cancer patients attending an outpatient pain and symptom clinic. J Palliat Care 1998;14(4):21–6.

[11] Tasaki K, Maskarinec G, Shumay DM, et al. Communication between physicians and cancer patients about complementary and alternative medicine: exploring patients' perspectives. Psychooncology 2002;11(3):212–20.

[12] Wyatt GK, Friedman LL, Given CW, et al. Complementary therapy use among older cancer patients. Cancer Pract 1999;7(3):136–44.

[13] Richardson MA, Sanders T, Palmer JL, et al. Complementary/alternative medicine use in a comprehensive cancer center and the implications for oncology. J Clin Oncol 2000;18:2505–14.

[14] Navo MA, Phan J, Vaughan C, et al. An assessment of the utilization of complementary and alternative medication in women with gynecologic or breast malignancies. J Clin Oncol 2004;22:671–7.

[15] Kao GD, Devine P. Use of complementary health practices by prostate carcinoma patients undergoing radiation therapy. Cancer 2000;88(3):615–9.

[16] Verhoef M, White M, Doll R. Cancer patients' expectations of the role of family physicians in communication about complementary therapies. Cancer Prevention and Control 1999;3(3):181–7.

[17] Robotin M, Penman A. Integrating complementary therapies into mainstream cancer care: which way forward? Medical Journal of Australia 2006;185(7):377–9.

[18] Berk LB. Primer on integrative oncology. Hematol Oncol Clin North Am 2006 Feb;20(1):213–31 Review.

[19] Cohen L, Cohen MH, Kirkwood C, Russell NC. Discussing complementary therapies in an oncology setting. Journal of the Society for Integrative Oncology 2007;5(1):18–24.

[20] SIO Mission. Society for Integrative Oncology. Available at: http://www.integrativeonc.org/index.php?scn=aboutus. Accessed October 21, 2007.

[21] Institute of Medicine: Cancer Care for the Whole Patient: Meeting Psychosocial Health Needs. The National Academies Press 2008 Prepublication available on line: http://www.nap.edu/catalog.php?record_id=11993. Accessed Feb 25, 2008.

[22] Hirshberg C, Barasch MI. Remarkable recovery. Reprint ed: Riverhead Trade; 1996.

Hematol Oncol Clin N Am 22 (2008) 581–617

HEMATOLOGY/ONCOLOGY CLINICS
OF NORTH AMERICA

Dietary Supplement Use in Cancer Care: Help or Harm

Mary L. Hardy, MD

Simms/Mann–UCLA Center for Integrative Oncology, University of California
at Los Angeles, 200 UCLA Medical Plaza, Suite 502 Los Angeles, CA 90095-9615, USA

The majority of cancer patients are using dietary supplements (DS) during all phases of cancer treatment, yet few topics are more controversial in integrative oncology. Despite increasing use by cancer patients, most conventional oncologists recommend complete avoidance of all supplements throughout most phases of cancer care [1]. This stance by oncologists limits disclosure of use of dietary supplements by patients and may, therefore, increase patients' risk. Furthermore, a closer look at the literature in this area does not support a blanket interdiction. Evidence of harm remains largely theoretic, while evidence of benefit in some cases may warrant active recommendation. This article looks at the evidence that exists both for and against use of dietary supplements during cancer care, to aid the practitioner in advising and managing care of patients using a wide variety of natural health products. Recommendations to maximize benefit and minimize harm while using DS are made.

Recent surveys confirm a high prevalence of complementary and alternative medicine (CAM) use, in some cases over 90% [2]. Even where general CAM use is low (23%), as in a recent survey of head and neck cancer patients, a large portion of CAM use involves herbs (47%) or herbal teas (23%) or vitamin-mineral preparations (12%) [3], products which conventional oncologists find particularly bothersome. CAM use increases after diagnosis [4], up almost eight times for herbs in one study [3], and remains high through out the spectrum of cancer care. High-risk women attending a genetic testing program were found to be using CAM at rates (53%) comparable to those reported in active treatment and use continued for at least one year, especially in breast cancer gene (BRCA)-1 positive patients [5,6]. Hospitalized cancer patients also have high rates of DS use (73% in previous 30 days) [7], and so do participants in National Institutes of Health (NIH) sponsored trials (63%) [8]. Use of biologically based CAM, defined as herbs, vitamins, and other dietary supplements, is still significant (34%), even in phase I trials of patients with advanced disease [9]. High rates of use of CAM (68%), with a large percentage using dietary

E-mail address: mhardy@mednet.ucla.edu

0889-8588/08/$ – see front matter
doi:10.1016/j.hoc.2008.04.012

supplements (80%), have also been reported in patients during radiation therapy [10]. Use of CAM modalities often continues long after completion of conventional oncology care [11].

Nondisclosure of CAM or DS use to medical providers is common throughout the spectrum of cancer care [10]. The majority (53%) of patients using dietary supplements during recent chemotherapy did not seek advice or guidance from a medical provider [7]. Disclosure, even if done, may be incomplete. In a recent survey, patients undergoing active, conventional therapy did disclose CAM use 57% of the time, but they were likely not to disclose all of the modalities they were using [2]. However, in situations where DS is part of routine medical care, such as head and neck cancer patients at an outpatient Veteran's Affairs clinic, disclosure is more common (62% disclosure of use). Patients are likely to hear about DS use from their physician (38%) and may even receive the supplement from the medical system directly (25%) [12]. Thus, involvement of the medical team in DS use facilitates full disclosure to the medical profession, which is crucial for optimal patient care.

Physicians' attitudes and knowledge about CAM therapies also influenced patient's likelihood of disclosure of use. Patients have cited expectations of a negative response or active opposition from their physicians as a reason to withhold disclosure [13], and this runs counter to their expectation for nonjudgment and support from their physician [14]. Many physicians do hold largely negative attitudes toward use of DS during cancer treatment [15], especially if CAM is perceived to be harmful or to be used as the sole treatment [16]. However, assessing harm maybe problematic, as many physicians have self-identified themselves as having little information about CAM cancer treatments [16] and their patients concur with this assessment [14].

In general, physicians do not share the same perception of benefit or possible benefit that their patients expect from CAM use [17]. They, like their patients, believe that CAM modalities can decrease side effects, but do not expect CAM to boost immunity or improve quality of life [17]. Strengthening the immune system is a common reason cited by patients, but not physicians, for DS use [18,19], as is a desire to decrease medication complications or relieve other symptoms, such as anxiety or depression [8,18]. While desire for a cure is less often stated as a reason, prevention of recurrence is a common reason for breast cancer patients to use CAM [19].

Furthermore, patients' and physicians' opinions diverge on what kind of evidence to use as a guide to CAM therapy. Patients place less emphasis on scientific evidence and rely on a much broader range of information, such as family, friends, and Internet sources [20]. Most oncologists place a much larger emphasis on scientific evidence [13], as they perceive complementary alternatives to be scientifically unproven [16]. However, when provided with online information, it has been shown that both patients and physicians have difficulty distinguishing high quality from low quality or biased information [21]. Therefore, in order for clinicians to be able to have a complete discussion with patients, they must first be aware of the existing clinical evidence.

RISKS OF ALTERNATIVE CANCER CARE

To fulfill the first caveat of clinical medicine, first do no harm, it is important to examine what evidence exists for risk associated with dietary supplement usage. Refusal of curative conventional treatment is often cited as a risk of CAM therapy by the conventional medical establishment [22]. Limited evidence does exist to support this concern. When alternative therapies were used as first-line treatment in a group of 33 women with breast cancer, early death and higher rates of recurrence were reported [23]. Furthermore, when tested in rigorous clinical trials, all "natural cancer cures" examined so far, such as shark cartilage [24,25], either have shown no benefit or, in the case of others such as laetrile [26], were found to be both ineffective and toxic. Fortunately, even for patients with advanced disease, most (88%) receive CAM care concurrently with conventional treatment [27] and it is the minority (8% in one study) who choose solely alternative cancer care [28]. Concurrent use of CAM with conventional care has generally shown no change in survival time [29]; however, some exceptions of both increased and decreased survival will be discussed below.

Risk from use of contaminated or adulterated dietary supplements has been suggested. When this occurs in products commonly used by cancer patients, patients can be exposed to unexpected ingredients that may themselves be toxic or may interfere with the action of pharmaceutic medications. In at least one case, substitution of one Chinese herb for another (*Stephania* for *Aristolochia*) caused acute nephrotoxicity and later development of genitourinary cancer [30]. Perhaps the most notorious example of a contaminated dietary supplement used by cancer patients is the herbal formula PC-SPES, which was found to contain warfarin, DES, and other substances [31,32]. These failures in quality control of botanical products have prompted concern in the public as well as the medical community. New dietary supplement manufacturing rules recently released by Food and Drug Administration are designed to address issues of dietary supplement quality [33].

In addition, relatively few herbs have toxic constituents that are not recommended for general use [34]. One serious but infrequent side effect of concern to oncologists is liver toxicity, especially given the inherently toxic nature of chemotherapeutic agents. Hepatotoxictiy has been reported for some common herbs, such as chaparral (*Larrea tridentate*), comfrey (*Symphytum officinale*), and kava (*Piper methysticum*) [35]. However, not all herbs with reports of hepatotoxicity have equally compelling evidence. For example, black cohosh (*Actea racemosa*), often used to treat menopausal symptoms—including those in women with or at high risk for breast cancer—has been alleged in a number of case reports to cause liver damage by at least two separate mechanisms, and has been subject to regulation by a number of international regulatory agencies [36]. However, in contrast, an expert conference that convened at the NIH in 2004 reviewed all of the available data and concluded that there was no demonstrated mechanism of action of hepatic injury for black cohosh, as well as insufficient evidence of toxicity, to warrant stopping or modifying clinical trials currently using black cohosh [37].

Herb-drug interactions, the form of adverse effect most often mentioned by oncologists, has been the subject of a number of reviews [38–42]. Despite these reviews and the concerns they raise, only two articles were identified that specifically tried to assess the degree of risk encountered by use of dietary supplements, including herbs, during cancer care [41,43]. Of the 76 chemotherapy patients surveyed to identify potentially negative chemotherapy-herb or vitamin interactions, only three of the patients were using herbs (St. John's wort or *Hypericum perforatumy* and garlic or *Allium sativum*) that might have affected the metabolism of their chemotherapy. In 318 chemotherapy patients who were also using herbal remedies [43], 11% took supplements in higher than recommended doses and potential interactions were identified in 12% of the patients ($n = 20$). Most of the warnings were given to lymphoma patients taking echinacea on the basis on potential adverse effects of immune stimulation. In neither study were confirmed interactions observed.

Concern for interactions is based on the ability of herbal products to affect the cytochrome P450 enzyme system that is crucial in the metabolism of a number of chemotherapeutic agents. Potential for interaction has also been raised with adenosine triphosphate binding-cassette transporters, such as P-glycoprotein, multidrug resistance associated protein-1, and breast cancer resistance protein [38]. Although herbal remedies have been shown to both up- and down-regulate the activity of a variety of P450 isozymes in screening tests, relatively few human clinical trials exist to validate these results [44]. One review by Sparreboom and colleagues [38] attempted to assess the likelihood of interaction of a number of common herbal agents with chemotherapy based on a wide variety of preclinical, animal, and human data. The investigators concluded that interactions with saw palmetto (*Serenoa repens*), cranberry (*Vaccinium macrocarpon*), black cohosh, milk thistle (*Silybum marianum*), and bilberry (*Vaccinium myrtillus*) were not expected, while specific cautions were made for garlic, ginkgo (*Ginkgo biloba*), soy (*Glycine max*), ginseng (*Panax ginseng*), valerian (*Valeriana officinalis*), and kava, largely on the basis of preclinical data.

Despite the high level of concern expressed in these cited reviews, only a handful of human pharmacokinetic studies were identified in the literature that directly assessed the effect of any herb on a chemotherapeutic agent. Ten breast cancer subjects took 600 mg of a proprietary garlic extract containing 3,600 mcg of allicin twice a day for days 5 to 17 of their chemotherapy cycle [45]. Docetaxel pharmacokinetics assessed before and after the administration of garlic showed no change in peak concentration, area under the curve (AUC), or half-life. Milk thistle (*Silybum marianum*) was tested in six cancer subjects taking irinotecan [46]. Four days before their second dose of irinotecan, subjects were given 200 mg of a commercially available milk thistle extract, standardized to 80% silymarin, three times a day. No significant effect on irinotecan clearance was noted despite a slight but borderline statistically significant decrease in the AUC. Serum concentrations of silybin, one of the constituents of milk thistle, were felt to be too low to be of concern for drug interactions.

Most of the reviews cited above agree that the herb with the strongest risk of clinically significant interactions is St. John's wort. Three human studies of the effect of St. John's wort on imatinib confirm the need for caution. Ten subjects, given 400 mg of imatinib before and after a treatment with 300 mg of St. John's wort three times a day [47] showed significant alterations in the pharmacokinetics of imatinib (32% reduction in AUC and a 29% reduction in maximal concentration). In a second study, 12 healthy subjects who were given 300 mg of a standardized proprietary St. John's wort product three times a day also had a significant increase in imatinib clearance (43%), as well as a 30% reduction in AUC [48]. Significant reductions were also noted in half-life and maximum concentrations. More worrisome was a small study of five cancer subjects taking irinotecan concurrently with 900 mg per day of St. John's wort extract. Plasma levels of SN-38, the active metabolite of irinotecan, were statistically significantly reduced (42%, $P = .033$) and, more significantly, myelosuppression was less during cotreatment as well [49]. However, in none of the studies was the composition of the St. John's wort extract described or independently confirmed by the investigators. In the case of St. John's wort this is particularly important, as most of the induction of the CYP450 enzymes is felt to be because of hyperforin, one constituent of St. John's wort extracts [50].

Interference with coagulation by herbs or other dietary supplements is of particular concern for oncology patients as they undergo surgery or other invasive procedures [51]. The investigators of this recent review postulate that antiplatelet actions, as well as interference with warfarin, could put cancer patients at risk. However, when commercially available extracts of ginkgo, garlic, Panax ginseng, St. John's wort, and saw palmetto were given to 10 healthy volunteers for 2 weeks, no effect on platelet activity was demonstrated [52]. Likewise, evidence of interaction of warfarin with herbs is based largely on case reports of variable (mostly poor) quality, which is not confirmed by pharmacologic studies [53].

Herbal therapies with estrogenic, androgenic, or progesterone-like activity are a theoretic concern for patients with hormone-sensitive cancers, particularly breast, ovarian, endometrial, or prostate cancers [54]. However, the majority of the literature on hormonal effects of herbs focuses on the estrogen activity of herbs commonly used for treating menopause. In preclinical trials, soy isoflavones and red clover extracts have been shown to have estrogenic activity of uncertain clinical significance for estrogen receptor-positive breast cancer patients [55]. Black cohosh, although mistakenly referred to as a phytoestrogen, does not appear to have estrogenic activity as tested in a variety of in vitro, animal, and human studies [56–58]. Neither does it appear to increase breast density [59]. The only formal safety study of a proprietary black cohosh extract (Klimadynon) was done in normal menopausal women [58]. Four hundred women were given 20 mg of herbal drug for 12 months under close observation. No increased uterine hypertrophy or heptatoxicity was noted during the trial. Breast density in the subset of women who had mammograms before and after the trial was lower, suggesting no toxic effect on breast tissue. Activity via serrotonergic neurons in the hypothalamus is thought to account for the clinical effect of black cohosh on vasomotor symptoms [60]. Therefore, the conservative recommendation to avoid consumption of high amounts of herbs with in vitro estrogenic activity does not apply to the use of black cohosh extract (BCE).

In summary, exposure has occurred from adulterated DS, such as PC-SPES, but few cases are noted. Evidence of hepatotoxicity of BCEs was not sufficient to warrant the interruption of ongoing clinical trials, nor is black cohosh a phytoestrogen. Despite widespread theoretic concern about herb-drug interactions, clinically significant interactions were only proved with St. John's wort. Observations from in vitro screening and animal studies need to be tested in human beings to confirm the presence or absence of clinically relevant interactions.

Evidence of interference with platelet function or warfarin activity was contradictory or absent for most herbs tested.

Antioxidants

Although antioxidant-rich foods are commonly associated with reduced risks of a variety of cancers, use of antioxidants, either singly or in formulas, as preventative agents for cancer has not been supported by large randomized trials [61]. In fact, at times antioxidant supplementation has been associated with harm when used preventatively [62]. Thus, use in conjunction with conventional therapy has remained a controversial area. Conventional practitioners usually have general prohibitions against use during chemotherapy or radiation [1]. However, a number of authorities have highlighted large amounts of preclinical and limited amounts of human clinical data in favor of use of at least some antioxidants [63–67]. Discussion of a limited selection of some of the key human clinical trials in this area will highlight key points in this debate.

Conventional clinicians cite fear of decreasing the effectiveness of conventional therapy as their major concern with the use of antioxidants during chemotherapy or radiation [1]. Some evidence exists for this concern. During a large randomized, double blind, placebo controlled trial of 540 patients with head and neck cancer undergoing radiation [68], subjects were given either placebo or a combination of antioxidants (400-IU alpha-tocopherol, 30-mg beta-carotene) daily throughout radiation therapy and for 3 years afterwards. Although acute side effects of radiation were significantly less in the antioxidant group, quality of life was not improved significantly, and the rate of local recurrence was higher in the supplemented group (odds ratio or OR 1.37; confidence interval or CI 0.93–2.02). Long-term follow-up of these subjects showed that at a median follow-up of 6.5 years, all-cause mortality was significantly higher in the treated group (hazard ratio or HR 1.38; CI 1.03–1.85) [69]. A historical cohort control study of 90 women who had taken large doses of beta-carotene, vitamin C, niacin, selenium, coenzyme Q10, and zinc during their conventional therapy were compared with matched controls [70]. Overall survival was the same for the two groups, but a trend toward reduction in disease-free survival was noted ($P = .08$). However, other studies did not confirm harm for patients undergoing chemotherapy. Although combination antioxidant therapy (6,100-mg ascorbic acid, 1,050-mg dl-alpha tocopherol, and 60-mg beta-carotene per day) did not improve the response rate of 136 advanced non-small cell lung cancer patients, neither did it diminish response rate or increase toxicity [71].

The greatest proponents of vitamin C use, Linus Pauling and his collaborators, suggested benefit from high-dose (10 gm) vitamin C in terminal patients who had exhausted all conventional options [72]. A cohort of 100 "untreatable" cancer patients who took 10 gm of vitamin C showed a greater mean survival of 300 days and a greater number of survivors after 1 year (24% versus 0.4%) than in a historical control group of 1,000 patients. Two subsequent randomized, controlled trials by other investigators failed to confirm benefit, though no significant toxicity was noted [73,74]. However, new reports of positive cases have lead researchers to open an NIH trial investigating further use of high-dose vitamin C [75,76].

Antioxidant use has also had reported benefit during active cancer treatment. Lower antioxidant intakes in a group of children with acute lymphocytic leukemia were associated with increases in adverse events during chemotherapy [77]. A decreased rate of chemotherapy-related nephro- and ototoxicity was only seen in the patients—supplemented with vitamins C, E, and selenium—who achieved the highest serum levels [78]. Experts have also cited preclinical and some limited human data to support the use of coenzyme Q10 to reduce the toxicity of anthrocyclin-based chemotherapy [79]. Benefit derived from antioxidant treatment for specific side effects of treatment are discussed in subsequent sections.

In summary, use of antioxidants during chemotherapy and radiation remains controversial. Most concerns are theoretic, although limited evidence for harm exists, mainly for vitamin E with head and neck patients. Experts cite large amounts of pre-clinical data and limited human data to support use of antioxidants, such as vitamin C, coenzyme Q10, and vitamin E for reduction of chemotherapy-related toxicity and possible tumor response in the case of vitamin C.

POTENTIAL BENEFITS OF DIETARY SUPPLEMENTS

A variety of natural products have shown benefit for cancer patients, either globally for overall quality of life, or for relief of specific symptoms associated with cancer treatment. To a lesser degree, especially with immunomodulatory agents, modification of tumor response, increases in disease-free interval, or prolonged survival have been seen. Certain substances will not be discussed in any detail, despite the fact that patients commonly use them. Compounds, such as the lectins from mistletoe (*Viscum album*) or a proprietary Japanese polysaccharide extract from shitake (*Lentinus edodes*) are usually delivered intravenously or parenterally, and therefore are not dietary supplements according to regulatory standards in the United States. Whole cannabis, extracts, and to a lesser degree isolated compounds from cannabis, have been noted to ameliorate a variety of symptoms in cancer patients, including pain, nausea, anorexia, and cachexia [80]. However useful many clinicians find the herbal form of this medicine, the legal ambiguity and challenges with standardization of dosage make use of this substance beyond the scope of this review.

Immune Modulation

Medicinal mushrooms and mushroom-derived polysaccharide preparations have been extensively studied as immune modulators and adjuvant agents in cancer treatment using in vitro and animal models with some human clinical trials as well [81–84]. In addition to improving quality of life or modifying tumor response, medicinal mushroom preparations have been shown to have beneficial effects on immune response, mainly in patients with solid, as opposed to hematologic, malignancies. One of the best studied preparations is a proprietary, protein-bound polysaccharide extract (PSK) of the medicinal mushroom, *Trametes versicolor,* also called *Coriolus versicolor.* PSK in a dose of 3 grams per day, was shown to decrease the serum level of the immunosuppressive acidic protein in a randomized trial of 207 stage II and III colorectal cancer patients, all of whom had conventional therapy [85,86]. After 5 years of follow-up, the treated patient group also had a greater percentage of 5-year disease free survival ($P = .038$) and a decreased relative risk of regional metastases (relative risk or RR 3.595; CI 1.518–8.518). These results are confirmed by a meta-analysis of three trials (reported in 10 articles) involving 1, 094 subjects with colorectal cancer [87]. Those who took PSK showed a significant improvement in overall survival (RR 0.71; CI 0.55–0.90; $P = .006$) and disease-free survival (RR 0.72; CI 0.58–0.90; $P = .003$) [87]. Benefit of PSK was also demonstrated in a meta-analysis of 8,009 gastric cancer patients from eight randomized, controlled trials with an increased survival (HR 0.88; CI 0.79–0.98; $P = .0180$) [88]. Specific clinical trials additionally cited an increase in disease-free survival rate for gastric cancer patients taking PSK with minimal toxicity [89]. A different extract of *Trametes versicolor* (Yunzhi) in combination with *Salvia militorrhiza* (Danshen) decreased the decline in absolute T-lymphocyte counts and preserved populations of T-helper and suppressor cells in a group of nasopharyngeal cancer patients receiving radiotherapy [90]. Immunologic parameters were also better in a group of 82 breast cancer patients after taking the Yunzhi/Danshen combination with an increase in T4 helper cells, an improvement in the CD4+/CD8+ ratio and an increase in B-lymphocytes [91].

A polysaccharide extract (active hexose correlated compound or AHCC) of a proprietary hybrid mushroom identified as *Basidiomycotina* has been tested in several human trials. Eleven advanced cancer patients (breast, ovarian, prostate, and multiple myeloma) were given 3 g per day of AHCC in an uncontrolled trial [92]. They showed a 2.5 times increase in natural killer cell (NK) activity, and 6 of 11 subjects were reported to have a tumor response. When either AHCC ($n = 34$) or placebo ($n = 10$) was given to advanced liver cancer patients, statistically significant increases in lymphocyte percentage ($P = .026$), albumin levels ($P = .000$), general physical health status ($P = .037$), and maintenance of activities of daily living ($P = .04$) were reported [93]. A highly statistically significant increase in survival was noted as well when compared with the control group ($P = .000$). A large cohort of 269 hepatocellular cancer subjects, after presumptively curative resection, was assigned prospectively after surgery to receive either 3-g of AHCC daily or control [94]. The treated group had a significantly longer disease-free interval (HR 0.639; CI 0.429–0.952; $P = .0277$), and increased overall survival (HR 0.421; CI 0.253–0.701; $P = .0009$).

A number of other medicinal mushrooms have also been tested in cancer patients, but the variable results seen may be caused in part by the phytochemical complexity and variety of extracts tested [83]. *Grifola* or *Polyporus umbellate,* also called Zhu ling in traditional Chinese medicine, was as effective as Bacillus Calmette-Guerin in preventing recurrence of bladder cancer following surgery, and was more effective than mitomycin C (34.9%, 35.1%, and 41.7% respectively) [95]. A proprietary extract (D-Fraction) of *Grifola frondosa,* also called Maitake, caused small changes in CD4+ and CD8+ counts while increasing NK cell activity in all 10 advanced cancer patients [96]. Oral polysaccharides from *Ganoderma lucidum,* also known as Ling zhi or Reishi, when given in a dose of 5.4 g per day for 12 weeks, improved the mitogenic reactivity to phytohemagglutinin, increased CD3, CD4, CD8, and CD56 lymphocyte counts, and increased NK activity, while elevating plasma concentrations of interleukin (IL)-2, IL-6, and gamma interferon, and decreasing tumor necrosis factor alpha and IL-3 in 46 subjects with a variety of advanced stage cancers [97,98]. However, a study in 30 advanced lung cancer patients showed marked variability in immune response to the Ganoderma extract, suggesting that certain subgroups of patients may be more responsive than others [99].

Finally, the use of an extract of the mushroom *Agaricus blazei,* given to 100 patients with gynecologic cancers (cervical, ovarian, or endometrial) undergoing conventional chemotherapy (carboplatin, etoposide, or taxol), showed a higher NK activity ($P < .002$), as well as a decrease in a variety of chemotherapy-related side effects, such as decreased appetite, alopecia, weakness, and emotional lability [100].

A proprietary fermented wheat germ extract standardized to methoxy-substituted benzoquinones (Avé or Avemar) has shown immunomodulatory and antitumor activity in a variety of preclinical studies and several human trials [101]. An open-label, matched-pair trial of pediatric cancer patients showed a decrease in the number of episodes of febrile neutropenia when compared with control (30 or 24.9% versus 46 or 43.4%) without any other differences in treatment [102]. Adult colorectal cancer patients undergoing conventional treatment were nonrandomly assigned to receive either usual care ($n = 104$) or usual care plus 9 g of Avé ($n = 66$) [103]. After 6 months of treatment, the Avé group had fewer new recurrences (3% versus 17%), new metastases (7.6% versus 23.1%), or death (12.1% versus 31.7%; all $P < .01$) with a significant increase in disease-free survival ($P = .018$) and overall survival ($P = .278$). Interim analysis of an ongoing randomized, controlled trial in Stage III melanoma patients ($n = 42$) receiving decarbazine chemotherapy shows an increased time-to-relapse for patients treated with Avé versus placebo (8.9 versus 4.2 months) without a decrease in relapse rate and with a larger percentage of treated patients free of disease at 1 year (54.5% versus 38.9%) [104].

Probiotics have also been used clinically for their immune modulating actions. In a group of 14 leukemia patients, pretreatment before chemotherapy continuing until the resolution of severe neutropenia (absolute neutrophil count > 1,000/μl) did not prevent the development of febrile neutropenia [105]. However, no evident toxicity of the therapy was identified. Pre- and postoperative supplementation with symbiotic treatment (*Lactobacillus casei*, *Bifidobacterium breve*, and galacto-oligosacchaides) was more efficacious than postoperative treatment alone in 81 biliary cancer patients undergoing hepatectomy [106]. Subjects in the pre- and postoperative treatment group had increased NK activity and lymphocyte counts, with decreased IL-6 preoperatively, and decreased white blood cell counts, IL-6, and C-reactive protein postoperatively. Postoperative infection rates were lower in the before and after group as well (12% versus 30%; $P < .05$). However, given the recent unexpected and as yet unexplained deaths in a trial using probiotics in patients with severe pancreatitis, caution may be advised [107].

In summary, medicinal mushroom extracts tested in a variety of cancers have shown benefit by improving immune parameters, increasing disease-free survival, and sometimes by enhancing tumor response. Data is strongest for the proprietary Coriolus extract PSK at a dose of 3 g per day, but positive data was also seen for other extracts, including AHCC, Maitake, and Agaricus. Benefit was also shown for a proprietary wheat germ extract Avé and probiotic preparations. No significant toxicities were reported in any of the trials reviewed, but adverse events in a recent probiotic trial (though not with cancer patients) require caution.

Stomatitis/Mucositis

Mucositis, a common side effect of both chemotherapy and local radiation, contributes significantly to patient morbidity through decreased quality of life and interference with proper nutrition. It is often the dose-limiting side effect for treatment [108,109]. A number of natural products have shown promise in preventing or alleviating oral mucositis, beginning with even the simplest therapy, such as ice chips (plain or flavored) or honey [110,111].

Glutamine is the DS that has been most often studied to prevent and treat oral mucositis resulting from either chemotherapy or radiation. The effects were strongest when head and neck patients were given intravenous glutamine (dose 0.4 g/kg per day) [112]. Clear improvements in chemotherapy-related mucositis were seen, with patients reporting a lower incidence of mucositis ($P = .035$), less severe mucositis ($P = .007$), and less pain ($P = .008$), as well as less need to insert a feeding tube ($P = .02$). Positive results were also seen in a number of trials using oral glutamine as a swish and swallow mouthwash. A phase I trial of oral glutamine (dose of 0.5 g/kg per day) was performed on

nine subjects with inflammatory breast cancer receiving neoadjuvant methotrexate followed by adriamycin [113]. Only one subject reported any mucositis
(grade I), with a good response to chemotherapy for eight of the nine subjects
and without any glutamine related toxicity. Similarly, a placebo controlled trial
of adults and children using glutamine (2 g/m^2 twice a day during chemotoxic
therapy) showed significant reductions in both severity ($P = .002$) and duration
of mucosisits pain (decreased by 4.5 days, $P = .0005$) [114]. Even subjects who
had pre-existing mucositis developed during an initial course of chemotherapy
responded well when 4-gm glutamine twice a day was given in subsequent sessions [115]. Twelve of 14 subjects decreased their maximum grade of mucositis
($P < .001$) and the total number of days with mucositis decreased by more than
two thirds ($P \geq .001$) following treatment.

Glutamine was also beneficial for children undergoing autologous bone marrow transplant when given at a dose of 1 g/m^2 four times a day throughout the
transplant and for 28 days afterwards [116]. Subjects reported less pain and
used morphine half as many days ($P = .005$). A second trial of children taking
2 g/m^2 to 4 g/m^2 of glutamine twice a day during stem cell transplant showed
decreased use of pain medication and fewer number of days using total paren-
teral nutrition as well [117]. In a retrospective chart review, adult breast cancer
patients ($n = 21$) undergoing autologous stem cell transplant following high-
dose paclitaxel showed similar positive results when given 24 g per day of
glutamine administered as a swish and swallow preparation around the clock
[118]. Treated women had fewer total days of narcotic pain relief and did
not require patient-controlled analgesia (PCA) morphine, while the untreated
group used PCA for 5.22 days. The women in the glutamine group also had
less oral ulceration and bleeding and were able to ingest liquids sooner than
the untreated group.

Radiation-induced mucositis in 17 head and neck cancer patients showed
a reponse to 16 gm of glutamine delivered four times a day by swish and
swallow [119]. After randomization to either glutamine or placebo, objective
evaluation showed a reduction of mean maximum grade of mucositis
($P = .0058$) and duration of mucositis at all grades (grade 1, $P = .0097$; grade 2,
$P = .0232$; grade 3, $P = .0168$). Subjective evaluations did not show the
same positive effect, except for the most severe mucositis (grade 3 or worse,
$P = .0386$). No changes in medication use or body weight were found.

However, despite the previous positive trials, a large phase III trial testing
oral glutamine with 5-fluorouracil (5-FU) chemotherapy did not show benefit
[120]. One hundred and thirty four subjects, randomized to receive 4 g of glutamine twice a day, were instructed to retain the glutamine mouthwash in their
mouths for only 10 seconds. No significant differences between groups were
seen regarding pain or severity of symptoms as assessed by either subjects or
physicians. The investigators speculated that the pretreatment with ice may
have blunted the expected positive effects of glutamine, but the short retention
time in the mouth was a possible factor in the poor response as well. In the final
analysis, it may be that glutamine is less effective for 5-FU chemotherapy, as an

additional small pilot study examining the effect of 16 g of glutamine for 8 days during treatment for gastrointestinal cancer also showed no benefit [121].

None of the glutamine studies reviewed demonstrated any toxicity, and the treatment was generally well tolerated. In one study where it was examined [116], glutamine did not increase the relapse rate, progression of malignancy, or incidence of graft-versus-host disease.

Vitamin E (formulation not reported), when given in a dose of 100 mg applied topically in the mouth of children who were receiving a variety of different chemotherapeutic agents, significantly improved their mucositis [122]. However, 16 children undergoing doxorubicin chemotherapy, given 800 mg of topical vitamin E or placebo using an N-of-1 study design, showed no advantage for vitamin E [123]. In a small trial of adults ($n = 18$) receiving a variety of different chemotheraputic regimens, swishing a vitamin E oil containing 400 mg/mL around the oral cavity twice a day resolved pre-existing mucositis in all but one subject [124]. Vitamin E also appears to have benefit in radiation-induced mucositis as well, as shown in a study where 54 patients with head and neck cancer undergoing radiation therapy were randomly assigned to rinse the oral cavity with either an oil containing 400 mg of vitamin E twice a day or an equivalent volume of evening primrose oil [125].

Zinc supplementation, 25 mg given three times a day during radiation therapy, delayed the development of grade 2 and reduced the number of grade 3 mucositis in a group of 50 head and neck cancer patients [126]. Concurrent administration of chemotherapy decreased the degree of benefit observed. In a similar group of subjects using a dose of 50 mg of zinc sulfate three times a day, not only was the incidence of mucositis less, but improvement after the development of mucositis started sooner in the treated group [127]. Two subjects of the treated group had no mucositis and none had grade 3 or 4 symptoms ($P = .05$).

Herbal therapy showed mixed results. Aloe vera mouthwash did show a non-statistically significant improvement in quality of life for 58 head and neck cancer patients during radiation treatment, but there was no difference in the number of patients with mucositis, the severity of symptoms, or weight [128]. Utility of chamomile extract mouthwashes was supported in some but not all of the trials. In an uncontrolled case series, a heterogeneous group of chemotherapy and radiation therapy subjects, treated with a commercial chamomile extract (Kamillosan), were reported to develop less mucositis if treated prophylactically and to heal faster if treated after symptoms developed [129]. A case report of a patient with severe mucositis following a methotrexate overdose reported resolution after rinsing with chamomile tea instead of using conventional treatments [130]. However, results from one large phase III study of 164 subjects receiving 5-FU and chamomile [131] did not show a benefit different from placebo. Unfortunately, the material used in this trial was not well described, so it is not possible to determine if the lack of response was because of a difference in materials.

A homeopathic remedy (Traumeel) containing *Arnica Montana* and other substances, when given as a mouthwash to 32 chemotherapy patients, significantly reduced the mean AUC of the stomatitis score ($P<.01$) compared with placebo [132]. In addition, more subjects in the treatment group did not develop any stomatitis (five versus one) and fewer subjects worsened during treatment with Traumeel (47% versus 93%).

Proteolytic enzymes decreased mucositis resulting from radiation therapy in a randomized open trial involving 100 head and neck patients [133]. From 3 days before until 5 days after radiation, subjects were given three tablets three times a day of a proprietary product containing 100 mg of papain, 40 mg of trypsin, and 40 mg of chymotrypsin. The maximum degree of mucositis was less in the treatment arm ($P<.001$). An additional smaller, randomized study of head and neck patients ($n = 50$) undergoing radiation therapy also demonstrated the effect of the same protolytic enzyme supplement regimen [109]. Decreases in severity of mucositis was noted, as well as decreased skin reactions, both highly statistically significant ($P<.001$). In addition, biopsies taken of the buccal mucosa before and after radiation therapy showed striking differences between the enzyme-treated and control groups.

In summary, simple interventions, such as ice, honey, and topical vitamin E oil can decrease stomatitis. The largest body of evidence supports the use of glutamine as an oral rinse, which is then swallowed to decrease stomatitis. Amounts of up to 30 g per day have been used without toxicity, but results with 5-FU chemotherapy were generally negative. Zinc, a proprietary homeopathic remedy, and proteolytic enzymes also showed benefit. Evidence for herbal therapies, such as aloe or chamomile mouthwashes, were mixed.

Intestinal Toxicity

Inflammation of the mucous membranes in the mouth is often associated with disruption of the gut mucosa, leading to gastrointestinal toxicity, such as leaky gut or diarrhea. In ten patients with chemotherapy-induced stomatitis, an oral challenge test demonstrated marked elevation in lactulose excretion when compared with 21 control subjects who did not have mucositis [134]. The degree of mucositis, not unexpectedly, is directly correlated with the severity of intestinal permeability (IP) [135]. Lactose intolerance increases during chemotherapy with 5-FU, and although it is reversible with the cessation of chemotherapy, it is accompanied by flatulence, diarrhea, and poor nutritional status [136]. Not unexpectedly, agents demonstrated to be helpful with stomatitis have also been tested for intestinal toxicity.

Glutamine showed benefit for chemotherapy-related intestinal toxicity in some studies [137]. A trial of 51 subjects receiving 5-FU chemotherapy with leucovorin rescue showed a significant correlation between the degree of stomatitis and abnormality of an oral challenge test for IP ($r = 0.898$, $P<.001$) [135]. Approximately half of the subjects in this trial were treated with 30 g per day of oral glutamine, while the control group received best supportive care. The glutamine-treated group showed a significantly lower IP score ($P<.001$) and had fewer subjects with a grade 2 to 4 mucositis than the control group (9% versus 38%; $P<.001$). A second trial of glutamine (18 g per day for

5 days before and until 15 days after chemotherapy) was compared with pla-cebo in 70 gastrointestinal cancer subjects receiving 5-FU [138]. Reduction in intestinal absorption and increase in permeability were significantly greater in the placebo arm ($P = .02$), while the incidence of diarrhea and use of lopera-mide tablets was decreased in the glutamine patients ($P = .09$ and $P = .002$, respectively). A small case series ($n = 6$) showed benefit using a proprietary oral glutamine product in metastatic colon cancer patients who had irinote-can-induced diarrhea unresponsive to loperamide and severe enough to require the suspension of therapy [139]. All patients restarted on chemotherapy with the addition of 10 g of glutamine three times a day beginning the day before irinotecan infusion and continuing until 4 days afterwards were able to tolerate full doses of chemotherapy.

When used in a randomized, controlled trial for breast cancer patients receiv-ing neo-adjuvant chemotherapy, glutamine given for a single round of chemo-therapy did significantly decrease IP ($P < .05$) but did not decrease the severity of stomatitis or diarrhea [140]. Perhaps, with a longer trial, differences in symp-toms would have followed the changes in permeability. However, breast cancer patients with advanced disease ($n = 33$) also did not decrease their diarrhea after taking 30 g of glutamine given in three divided doses for 8 days during the interval between doxifluridine chemotherapy [141].

Used in conjunction with pelvic radiation therapy, glutamine did not prevent gastrointestinal toxicity in a trial of 129 subjects with gynecologic cancers [142]. Subjects were randomly assigned to receive either a relatively low dose of glu-tamine (4 g twice a day) or placebo from the onset of radiation until 2 weeks after completion of the course of treatment. There were no differences between groups with respect to high-grade diarrhea (20% versus 19%) or maximum number of stools per day (5.1 versus 5.2).

Despite mixed evidence for efficacy, there was no evidence of decreased re-sponse to chemotherapy. In the Li and colleagues [140] study, the neoadjuvant breast cancer patients did not show any adverse effect on tumor response, with no change in tumor size, the Ki 67 index, or proliferating cell nuclear antigens (PCNA). Similarly, the Bozzetti and colleagues [141] trial of advanced breast cancer patients showed similar response rates to chemotherapy between the glutamine and the placebo groups (21% versus 28%).

Probiotics have been used to decrease gastrointestinal toxicity resulting from both chemotherapy and radiation. Colorectal cancer patients receiving one of two 5-FU chemotherapy regimens were also randomized to receive either *Lactobacillus rhamnosus* GG at a dose of 1 to 2 × 10(10) organisms or 11 g of guar gum per day [143]. Subjects receiving the probiotic had fewer episodes of high-grade diarrhea (22 versus 37%, $P = .027$) and less abdominal discom-fort. They also needed less hospital care and had fewer reductions in chemo-therapy because of bowel toxicity. No toxicity was noted with the *Lactobacillus* therapy. A different *L. rhamnosus* strain, also called Antibiophilus, was given in a randomized, double-blind fashion to 206 subjects receiving abdominal and pelvic radiation [144]. Subjects receiving the probiotic had fewer bowel movements with a trend toward statistical significance $(P < .1)$, with a significantly better consistency of fecal material $(P < .05)$. In addition, subjects reported fewer episodes of high-grade diarrhea in the probiotic group. Similar benefits were seen for 190 subjects receiving adjuvant radiotherapy for sigmoid, rectal, or cervical cancer [145]. Subjects received three times a day either a packet of a proprietary blend of eight species of lyophilized bacteria (VPL#3) containing 450 billion live bacteria per gram or placebo. The treated subjects reported significantly less diarrhea $(P < .001)$, lower grades of diarrhea when they did develop it $(P < .001)$, and fewer bowel movements (4.6 versus 12.3; $P < .05$). Two subjects in the placebo group needed to stop therapy because of gastrointestinal side effects, while none in the treatment group modified therapy on this basis. No treatment-related toxicity was reported from the probiotic group. A larger cohort of similar subjects $(n = 490)$ from the same research team, using the same intervention, showed similar benefit [146]. Treated subjects showed a lower incidence of radiation-induced diarrhea (32% versus 52%; $P < .001$), less severe high grade diarrhea (1% versus 33%; $P < .001$), and fewer number of bowel movements (15 versus 5; $P < .05$). Again, the therapy was well tolerated.

In summary, glutamine in similar doses as used for stomatitis showed more mixed results for prevention or treatment of chemotherapy and radiation-induced intestinal toxicity. Again, no evidence for significant toxicity was found. Probiotics given concurrently with chemotherapy or radiation decreased the severity of diarrhea without reports of toxicity. Theoretic cautions with probiotics were noted previously.

Neuropathy

Peripheral neuropathy is a potentially debilitating side effect caused by a number of chemotherapeutic agents, especially the platinum-based drugs and taxanes. Several dietary supplements have shown promise in ameliorating chemotherapy-induced neuropathy in human clinical trials [147].

In a nonrandomized, controlled clinical trial, patients receiving high-dose paclitaxel $(n = 45)$ were given either usual care $(n = 12)$ or glutamine $(n = 33)$ at a dose of 10 g, three times a day for 4 days starting 24 hours after chemotherapy [148]. The glutamine-treated group showed a statistically significant decrease in the severity of sensory neuropathy both for dysesthesia and numbness $(P < .05)$, as well as better motor function with a lower incidence and severity of motor weakness $(P = .04)$ and less disturbance in gait $(P = .016)$, resulting in less interference with the activities of daily living for the glutamine group $(P = .001)$. A second nonrandomized, controlled trial in 46 subjects receiving high-dose paclitaxel showed that the glutamine-treated group $(n = 17)$, after an average of 32 days of treatment, had significantly less weakness $(P = .02)$, better vibratory sensation $(P = .04)$, and less toe numbness $(P = .004)$ [149]. Nonstatistically significant improvements were seen in compound motor action potential and sensor nerve action potential measurement in the treatment group. Eighty-six metastatic colon cancer patients in a pilot study of the effect of glutamine on the neurotoxicity of oxaliplatin/5-FU chemotherapy showed that glutamine ($n = 44$), given at a dose of 15 g twice a day for the first 7 days of chemotherapy, reduced the incidence of moderate grade neuropathy after two (17% versus 39%), four (5% versus 18%), and six cycles (12% versus 32%) of treatment [150]. The benefit continued to accrue to the glutamine group despite a lack of difference in elecrophysiologic abnormalities, which translated into less interference with activities of daily living (17% versus 41%) and less reduction in chemotherapy (7% versus 27%) because of neuropathy. There was no difference in response to chemotherapy or survival between the two groups.

Vitamin E (alpha-tocopherol), given concurrently with platinum or taxane-based chemotherapy, has shown benefit in preventing chemotherapy-related neuropathy. A small, randomized trial enrolled 47 subjects to either usual care or to 300 mg of alpha-tocopherol twice a day throughout treatment with cisplatin chemotherapy, and for 3 months after completion [151]. Of the 27 subjects who completed the trial, the vitamin E group ($n = 13$) showed a decreased incidence (31% versus 86%; $P < .01$) as well as decrease in severity ($P < .01$) of neurotoxicity. No differences were seen in tumor weight, growth delay, or survival between the two groups. An additional three reports on the use of vitamin E to reduce chemotherapy toxicity were found [152–154]. They were all performed by the same research group and may represent multiple reports on the same patient population, so they will be discussed in aggregate. Subjects were given cisplatin, paclitaxel, or a combination of both, usually for six cycles, and were also randomly assigned to either a usual care group or to receive 600 mg of vitamin E per day during chemotherapy and for 3 months afterwards. The incidence of neuropathy was less in the treated group ($P = .019$–0.03) and the relative risk of developing neurotoxicity was found to be significantly higher in the control group (RR = 0.25–2.51). No adverse events or death were attributed to vitamin E use.

In summary, glutamine in doses of up to 30 g per day decreased the incidence and severity of chemotherapy-related neuropathy. Despite previously cited risks from vitamin E, doses of 300 mg to 600 mg decreased neuropathy during chemotherapy without any evidence of adverse events in these trials.

Nausea

Ginger has been suggested to treat nausea from multiple causes, including those associated with cancer treatment, although the literature in this area is more limited. Subjects ($n = 120$) undergoing major gynecologic surgery for malignant conditions were randomized to receive either 1 g of ginger or placebo an hour before surgery [155]. A visual analog scale of nausea and incidence of vomiting were lower in the treated group throughout the first 24 hours after surgery. No adverse events were reported. An early trial suggested that ginger could also help relieve nausea associated with 8-methoxsalen chemotherapy, but this trial was not randomized [156]. The ability of ginger to reduce acute and delayed nausea associated with cisplatin-based chemotherapy was tested in a randomized, double-blind placebo-controlled crossover trial [157]. Forty-eight subjects with gynecologic malignancies treated with cisplatin therapy were randomized to receive either placebo or 1 g per day of ginger orally for the first 5 days of the chemotherapy cycle on the first day, and metaclopramide daily for the next 4 days. All subjects received standard antiemetics on the first day. After the first cycle, patients were crossed over to the alternate protocol. Ginger performed as well as metaclopramide for delayed nausea with less restlessness, but the addition of ginger to conventional antiemetics did not improve acute efficacy.

In summary, ginger in doses as low as 1 gram of powdered herb per day showed benefit by reducing chemotherapy-related nausea. No serious adverse events were seen and ginger had fewer side effects than metaclopramide, a standard drug used for the same indication.

Radiation-Induced Dermatitis

Skin changes that occur commonly during radiation therapy usually don't limit treatment, but they do contribute to morbidity for patients. Unfortunately, most natural products tested to relieve radiation-induced dermatitis, with a few exceptions, did not show benefit. Aloe vera is one of the most commonly used topical agents used by cancer patients for radiation therapy-induced burns. Clinical trials and systematic reviews have not, unfortunately, been able to confirm a robust benefit [158]. A small controlled trial added aloe vera (product composition not fully described) to usual skin prophylaxis in patients receiving radiation therapy [159]. The aloe vera was applied "liberally to the [treated] area at various intervals throughout the day." At higher doses of radiation ($>$2,700 cGy), aloe treatment delayed the onset of skin changes by 2 weeks, from 3 to 5 weeks. A larger phase III trial ($n = 194$) of breast cancer patients receiving radiation to the chest wall were randomized to apply either 98% pure aloe vera gel or an inert control gel to the treated area twice a day throughout treatment [160]. Groups, identical at the start of the experiment based on age, surgery, radiation dose, and skin type still showed no difference after treatment. The only toxicities noted were three cases of aloe allergy and one allergic reaction in the control group. A second unblinded study of 108 women, reported in the same article, compared aloe vera gel to no therapy and again, there was no discernable difference between the two groups with respect to dermatitis [160].

Other herbal preparations have shown some benefit. A controlled clinical trial comparing a proprietary chamomile skin cream to almond oil, a standard therapy in the center conducting the trial, was undertaken in 48 women with breast cancer [161]. They were randomly assigned to apply either the chamomile cream or the almond oil to the area above and below the scar. Although the results were not statistically significant, the researchers concluded that chamomile cream delayed the onset of dermatitis and had a mitigating effect on severity. Allergic reactions occurred in two chamomile-treated patients and one almond oil patient. A large phase III clinical trial tested the efficacy of a calendula or trolamine in preventing grade II or higher dermatitis in breast cancer patients during radiation [162]. Subjects ($n = 254$) were randomized to apply either to a proprietary calendula homeopathic lotion or trolamine to the skin at least twice a day throughout the course of radiation. The incidence of grade II or higher dermatitis was significantly less in the calendula group (41% versus 63%; $P< .001$). Subjects reported greater satisfaction with the calendula lotion as well, despite rating it as being harder to apply.

In summary, topical aloe did not show consistent benefit in preventing or treating radiation dermatitis. One large trial of a calendula homeopathic lotion showed that it was effective and well tolerated in preventing skin changes because of radiation therapy.

Cachexia

Several systematic reviews and meta-analyses have examined the role of omega-3 fatty acids in preventing cancer-related cachexia [163–165]. The strictest of the three only includes five studies and suggests that the literature is insufficient to judge whether eicosapentaenoic acid (EPA) is superior to placebo in treating cachexia. However, two other reviews with broader inclusion criteria come to different conclusions. When the results of an analysis that included all controlled trials was presented to a panel of experts, they concluded that patients with advanced malignancies of the pancreas and upper digestive tract accompanied by weight loss benefited from oral supplementation with omega-3 fatty acids (ω3FA) [164]. These benefits included increases in weight and appetite, especially if ω3FA (a combination of EPA and docosahexaenoic acid or DHA) were given in a dose of 1.5 g per day. Heterogeneity existed in the composition of the ω3FA supplements and the mode of delivery, but lower fat formulas appeared to be better tolerated. Looking specifically at radiation therapy patients, pooling of available data suggested that use of ω3FA-rich nutritional formulas lead to a significant increase in dietary intake of approximately 380 kcal per day when compared with routine care [165]. A closer examination of some individual studies provides clinically useful information.

A phase I trial in 22 subjects with advanced disease established the upper limit of tolerance for oral fish oil capsules as 0.3 g/k per day [166]. The capsules tested contained 378-mg EPA and 249-mg DHA per gram of fish oil, suggesting that the maximal dose of ω3FAs for a 70-kg man was 13.1 g per day (0.19 g/kg). Doses were limited by gastrointestinal toxicity, mainly diarrhea, without any reports of serious adverse effect on coagulation or tumor response. However, for acceptable compliance over time, a much lower dose of fish oil, approximately 6 g per day, was found to be the maximum tolerated in a trial of subjects with advanced lung cancer [167].

Burns and colleagues [168] suggested that a relatively high dose of EPA is required for effect. In a follow-up phase II trial they tested a dose (7.5 g of EPA for a 70-kg patient or 0.11 g per day), which was approximately half of the maximally tolerated dose in their prior phase I trial. Only 6 subjects showed any weight gain, but the majority of the enrolled subjects did show stabilization of their weight (24 of 36 subjects). The investigators noted that this dose was double the dose tested in most other phase III trials and may have accounted for poor effect seen in some published studies.

Fish oil has also been tested in combination with other conventional medications. When combined with megase, the conventional treatment for cancer-related anorexia, no additional benefit was seen by adding 2.18 g of EPA per day [169]. However, combining fish oil (2 g three times a day) with celecoxib (200 mg twice a day) showed significantly greater improvements in appetite, fatigue, body weight, and muscle strength than with fish oil alone in a small group of subjects with advanced lung cancer [167]. C-reactive protein levels were also significantly lower in the combination group, suggesting that fish oil, as well as celecoxib, may have their benefit through interference with inflammation. A complex intervention involving a number of products (300-mg alpha lipoic acid; 400-mg vitamin E; 30,000-IU vitamin A, 500-mg vitamin C; omega-3 fatty acids) as well as the pharmaceuticals medroxyprogesterone (500 mg) and 200-mg celecoxib daily showed significant improvement on two different measures of quality of life [170].

In summary, fish oil, rich in ω3FAs, showed benefit in stabilization or reduction of cancer-related cachexia, but relatively high doses were required for effect. Weight stabilized or improved at 7.5-g EPA or fish oil. Combining fish oil with cyclooxygenase-2 inhibitors but not megase improved efficacy. Adherence was limited by gastrointestinal toxicity (diarrhea and nausea).

Lymphedema

Edema following conventional cancer care can be very problematic for patients and difficult to treat. Although a trial with vitamin E and pentoxifylline did not show benefit [171], one randomized trial with selenium selenite did reduce the upper extremity edema and improve the function of breast cancer patients enrolled in a decongestive physical therapy program [172]. Subjects were given 1,000 mcg of selenium selenite for the first week of the trial, 300 mcg for next 2 weeks, and then took a maintenance dose of 100 mcg for 3 months. A positive effect of selenium selenite was also reported in 10 of 12 patients with lymphedema following breast cancer treatment [173].

In addition, a number of small studies using flavinoid-rich preparations have also shown benefit. A proprietary gingko formula was given to 48 women with upper extremity edema following breast cancer treatment, and showed a reduction in the symptoms of limb heaviness as well as an increase in lymph migration speed [174]. Following a successful pilot using a proprietary micronized flavinoid fraction [175], a larger randomized controlled trial was performed on 104 women with lymphedema following breast cancer treatment [176]. Despite showing improvements in lymphatic migration speed by scintography, subjects reported a nonstatistically significant improvement in symptom relief. Greatest benefit accrued to the more severely affected women. A second small randomized, placebo-controlled pilot by a different research group also showed benefit in postmastectomy patients with edema when given 500 mg twice a day of a micronized, purified flavinoid fraction [177]. Fifty seven patients treated with either a proprietary formula of ruscus and hesperidin methyl chalcones or placebo for 3 months showed a 12.9% reduction in limb volume in the treatment group ($P = .009$) [178]. Conversely, a randomized phase II trial of 66 women with breast induration following radiation did not show benefit from a grape seed extract at a dosage of 100 mg three times a day for 6 months [179].

Head and neck patients also develop bothersome edema and tissue induration during radiotherapy, and selenium has shown some benefit in clinical trials [180]. Thirty-six patients with edema after radiotherapy, including 20 who had endolaryngeal edema with stridor and dyspnea, were included in an uncontrolled trial [173,181]. Patient self-assessment of symptoms on a visual analog scale showed statistically significant improvement after treatment ($P < .05$). Head and neck cancer patients ($n = 20$), given 1,000 mcg of selenium selenite per day orally or intravenously for three weeks in the perioperative period, had reduction in edema [182].

In summary, selenium at a dose of 300 mcg per day (perhaps with a loading dose of 1,000 mcg for 1 week), decreased lymphedema in breast and head and neck cancer patients without reported toxicity. A number of proprietary flavinoid-rich extracts, such as ginkgo or bioflavinoid extracts, also improved symptoms with noticeable side effects.

Fatigue

Fatigue, one of the most common and debilitating side effects of conventional cancer care, has been ameliorated to only a limited degree by dietary supplements. In fact, a randomized, double-blind trial of a common proprietary multiple vitamin did not relieve fatigue in 40 breast cancer patients undergoing radiation therapy [183]. More promising was a pilot study of cancer patients with fatigue and carnitine deficiency [184]. After 1 week of supplementation, 13 of 15 subjects increased total and free carnitine along with decreases in fatigue, as measured by Brief Fatigue Inventory scale, and Karnofsky performance status. Similar responses were seen in a group of patients receiving cisplatin or isofosfamide chemotherapy [185]. After 1 week of 4 g of carnitine daily, 45 of 50 subjects with abnormal fatigue significantly improved ($P < .001$) and they maintained their gains through the next cycle of chemotherapy. Longer administration of L-carnitine was tested in a small ($n = 12$), uncontrolled clinical trial. Subjects with advanced disease undergoing cytotoxic chemotherapy were given 6 g per day of L-carnitine with a measurable improvement in fatigue and quality of life [186]. A formal phase I/II study was undertaken to assess the safety of carnitine supplementation [187]. Subjects with advanced cancer, significant fatigue, and compromised activity (Karnofsky performance status of greater than or equal to 50) were enrolled in a dose-ranging study of L-carnitine. Of the screened patients, 77% (29 of 38) had deficient levels of carnitine at baseline. Of the 21 subjects who participated in the study, 17 raised their carnitine levels to normal with oral supplementation. Dosing started at 250 mg per day and increased to a maximum of 3,000 mg per day in divided doses. No toxicities were observed and in the 17 responders, a dose response effect was seen for carnitine levels and fatigue scores ($P = .01$). Positive effects were more likely at higher dose ranges.

In summary, DS for cancer-related fatigue were generally ineffective. Carnitine supplementation (up to 3,000 mg per day) decreased fatigue and improved quality of life in carnitine-deficient patients during chemotherapy.

Vasomotor Symptoms

Vasomotor symptoms related to natural menopause or cancer therapy, especially in younger women, cause significant morbidity for high-risk patients unable to take estrogen replacement therapy or for breast cancer survivors on hormonal therapy. Black cohosh extract has been suggested as a possible therapy to moderate vasomotor symptoms in this group.

Not all clinical trials have shown benefit in women with breast cancer, but some of the differences in response may be because of variations in the material used or the duration of the trial, as well as large, variable placebo effects commonly seen in menopausal studies. Breast cancer patients, after completion of conventional therapy (59 on tamoxifen; 26 on no hormonal therapy), were enrolled in a randomized, placebo-controlled trial of 8 weeks duration [188]. Both groups (placebo and proprietary black cohosh extract of Remifemin, 40 mg per day) showed similar improvements in number and intensity of hot flashes. The same extract studied in a small pilot study ($n = 21$) at the same dose showed a 56% reduction in hot flash frequency at the end of a 4-week open-label trial [189]. A follow-up phase III trial based on this pilot did not show any benefit [190]. However, the study medication was not the previously used proprietary product, but an extract prepared by the study team, which attempted to approximate the composition of the original. Perhaps this contributed to the marked difference in outcome of the two trials. Finally, a different proprietary product (Klimadynon) was used in the largest and longest study, an open-label trial of 136 women with breast cancer who had completed all conventional therapy and were being maintained on tamoxifen [191]. Two-thirds of the women were given a proprietary BCE (20 mg of herbal drug per day) for 12 months. At the end of that time, almost half of the intervention group were free of hot flashes, with severe hot flashes being reported in only 24% of the treatment group versus 74% of the control group ($P < .01$). No serious adverse events were reported.

Far from being detrimental to women with respect to breast cancer risk, two case controlled studies recently published suggest a protective effect. A case-controlled study of menopausal women identified 949 breast cancer patients and 1,524 controls [192]. Women who took BCE had more than a 50% reduction in risk of developing breast cancer (adjusted OR of developing breast cancer of 0.47; CI 0.27–0.82). Protective effects were also seen in a cohort of breast cancer subjects examined in a retrospective cohort study [193]. The effect of BCE on disease free survival was tested in 1,102 breast cancer survivors who took BCE, compared with a control group who did not. Use of BCE, after correction for other confounders such as tamoxifen use, showed a prolongation of disease-free survival. After 2 years, the group without BCE had a 14% recurrence rate. It took the BCE group until 6.5 years to achieve the same level of recurrence. The hazard ratio for recurrence was 0.83 (CI 0.69–0.99). These data suggest that BCE is unlikely to cause an increase risk of breast cancer recurrence and may in fact provide protection from recurrence.

In summary, proprietary BCEs have shown variable efficacy. Current safety data does not suggest estrogenic activity for BCEs, nor serious risk of hepatotoxicity. Preliminary cohort data suggests that BCEs may modify risk of recurrence.

Treatment of Pre-cancerous or Specific Lesions

Although dietary supplements are not appropriate as primary treatment in cancer, interesting data are emerging regarding selective use in treating premalignant lesions, some early cancers usually treated with watchful waiting, or specific treatment-resistant cancers. Fifty-nine subjects with oral leukoplakia were treated with either 3 gm of tea or placebo [194]. After 6 months, the treatment group showed a decrease in lesion size (38% versus 10% of subjects) and a lower number of micronucleated exfoliated cells (5.4 per 1,000 cells versus 11.3 per 1,000 cells; $P < .01$). Clinical improvement, decreases in micronuclei frequency in exfoliated cells, and reduction in chromosome abnormality was also seen in men treated orally with black tea in second study after 1 year of treatment [195].

High-grade intraepithelial neoplasia of the prostate (HG-PIN) has responded well to oral administration of a green tea extract [196]. When given 600 mg per day of a high catechins extract (total catechins 75.7%) or placebo for 1 year, progression to frank prostate cancer was 30% in the placebo group and only 3% in the treated group. Total prostate specific antigen (PSA) did not change, and men with symptomatic benign prostatic hyperplasia reported symptom reduction. Pomegranate juice (8 oz of concentrate, POM Wonderful variety), when given to men with a rising PSA following surgery or radiation, increased the mean PSA-doubling time from 15 months to 54 months ($P < .001$) without reports of adverse events [197]. When given a dietary supplement containing soy, lycopene, silymarin, and antioxidants (formulary details not given) following surgery or radiation for 10 weeks, 49 men showed an increase of PSA-doubling time from 445 days to 1,150 days, along with significant decreases in PSA slope ($P = .03$) [198].

Hormone-resistant or refractory prostate cancer (HRPC) can be very difficult to treat and there is interest in finding less toxic alternatives. A small trial ($n = 20$) studied the effect of 10 mg per day for 3 months of lycopene supplementation (Lycored brand) in patients with metastatic HRPC [199]. Tumor responses were seen (5% complete; 30% partial; 50% stable; 15% progression) in some of the study group, but the majority of patients (62%) were able to reduce amount of daily analgesics used, showing an improvement in bone pain. No toxicity from the lycopene supplementation was noted. Furthermore, the

Table 1
Safety dietary supplements in cancer care

Supplement	Action	Reference
Alternative therapy for sole treatment of breast cancer	Early death and higher rates of recurrence	[23]
Garlic extract with docetaxel	No change in pharmacokinetics	[45]
Milk thistle with irinotecan	No change in pharmacokinetics	[46]
St. John's wort with imatinib and irinotecan	Reduced serum levels	[47–49]
Black cohosh extracts	No evidence estrogenic activity	[56–60]
Beta-carotene and alpha tocopherol in head and neck patients during radiation	Increased rate local recurrence and high all cause mortality at 6.5 years	[68]
Vitamin C, beta-carotene, alpha tocopherol in non-small cell lung cancer patients during chemotherapy	No change in response rate; no increase in toxicity	[71]
Glutamine in bone marrow transplant	Did not increase relapse rate, progression of malignancy or incidence of graft versus host disease	[116]
Glutamine in breast cancer patients	No adverse effect on tumor response	[140,141]
Vitamin E in variety of solid tumors with cisplatin chemotherapy	No change in tumor response or survival	[151]

addition of lycopene (4 mg per day) to orchiectomy was also shown to improve the outcome of men with metastatic hormone-responsive cancer [200]. PSA, lower in the lycopene group from 6 months, was significantly lower by 2 years (3.01 ng/mL versus 9.02 ng/mL; $P < .001$), and almost twice as many lycopene treated subjects had a complete response (78% versus 40%). Formulation of the lycopene product may affect response, as a clinical trial of 46 subjects with HRPC did not respond to 15 mg of lycopene supplementation given twice a day in the form of tomato paste or juice [201].

In summary, preliminary data suggests that selected dietary supplements may play a role in treating precancerous lesions, such as tea for leukoplakia. Early cancerous lesions of the prostate (HG-PIN) that are conventionally treated by watchful waiting, may also benefit from the use of green tea extracts, pomegranate concentrates, or complex dietary supplements. The use of lycopene for hormone refractory prostate cancer showed mixed results. However, because of its low toxicity, it might be worth trying in doses of 4 mg to 30 mg per day.

SUMMARY

To meet the needs of the large number of cancer patients who are using DS, physicians and other health care providers must adopt strategies that encourage

Table 2
Efficacy dietary supplements in cancer care

Supplement	Action	Reference
Vitamin C, E, and selenium in chemotherapy patients	Decreased rate nephro and ototoxicty	[78]
Coenzyme Q10 with anthrocycline chemotherapy	Decrease cardiotoxicity	[79]
Trametes versicolor extract in variety of solid malignancies	Increased percentage of 5-year disease-free survival; decreased relative risk of regional metastases; improvement in overall survival	[85–89]
Basidiomycotina extract in variety of solid malignancies	Increased NK cell activity; improvement in activities of daily living (ADL); longer disease-free survival interval	[92–94]
Grifola umbellatae in bladder cancer	More effective than mitomycin C in preventing recurrences after surgery	[95]
Agaricus blazei extract in variety gynecologic cancers with chemotherapy	Increased NK cell activity and decreased general symptoms	[100]
Fermented wheat germ extract in pediatric cancer patients	Decreased episodes of febrile neutropenia	[101]
Fermented wheat germ extract in colorectal or melanoma cancer patients	Lower incidence of new disease, new metastases, or death; increased time to relapse	[102,103]
Probiotics in biliary cancer patients undergoing surgery; colorectal cancer patients undergoing chemotherapy; patients receiving abdominal and pelvic radiation	Lower postoperative infection rates; decreased gastrointestinal toxicity (diarrhea) with less hospital care and less reduction in chemotherapy; decreased incidence of diarrhea	[106,143–146]
Glutamine in variety of cancer patients undergoing chemotherapy and radiation	Decreased rates and severity of mucositis, neuropathy, and intestinal toxicity; decreased use of pain medication in stomatitis patients; improved nutrition in stomatitis patients; improved ADL in neuropathy patients	[112–119, 137–139, 148–150]
Vitamin E topically in children undergoing bone marrow transplant; in adults undergoing chemotherapy or radiation to head and neck area	Improved stomatitis	[122,124,125]
Zinc in head and neck patients during radiation therapy	Improved stomatitis	[126,127]

(continued on next page)

Table 2
(continued)

Supplement	Action	Reference
Chamomile extract as mouthwash in chemotherapy and radiation	Improved stomatits sometimes	[129,130]
Homeopathic remedy including Arnica montana in chemotherapy	Improved stomatitis	[132]
Proteolytic enzymes in head and neck patients with radiation	Improved stomatitis	[109,133]
Vitamin E orally in variety of cancers during cisplatin chemotherapy; patients with cisplatin and paclitaxel chemotherapy	Decreased rate of neuropathy	[151–154]
Ginger postoperatively in surgical cancer patients; with MOPP chemotherapy; with cisplatin chemotherapy	Decreased nausea	[155–157]
Calendula homeopathic lotion in radiation therapy	Decreased dermatitis	[162]
Chamomile skin cream	Decreased dermatitis	[161]
Fish oil in patients with cancer induced cachexia	Increased dietary intake, maintenance of weight, decreased fatigue	[163–170]
Selenium selenite in breast cancer and head and neck cancer patients	Decreased lymphedema	[171–173, 180–182]
Ginkgo in breast cancer patients	Decreased lymphedema	[174]
Variety of high flavinoid extracts	Decreased lymphedema	[175–179]
Carnitine in cancer patients following chemotherapy; benefit most pronounced in patients with carnitine deficiency	Decreases fatigue	[184–187]
Black cohosh extracts in breast cancer patients with menopausal symptoms	Decreases vasomotor symptoms in some trials	[189,191]
Green or black tea in leukoplakia	Improved abnormality	[194,195]
Green tea extract in high-grade intraepithelial neoplasia of the prostate without conventional therapy	Decreased progression to frank prostate cancer	[196]
Pomegranate juice in prostate cancer patients with rising PSA after radiation or surgery	Increased PSA-doubling time	[197]
Soy in complex formula in prostate cancer patients with rising PSA after radiation or surgery	Increased PSA-doubling time	[198]
Lycopene in hormone refractory prostate cancer; in hormone responsive patients following orchiectomy	Limited clinical response in some patients; Improved clinical response	[199–201]

Box 1: Recommendations to maximize gain and minimize risk in use of dietary supplement during cancer care

Encourage full disclosure from patients.

Assist patients to establish reasonable goals.

Develop a nuanced message about dietary supplement use.

Develop knowledge base regarding dietary supplements.

Favor dietary supplements from well-known, reputable companies.

Favor simpler over more complex dietary supplements.

Favor products that have been tested in human clinical trials.

Ask to see the actual products that patients are using.

Ask to see the resources patients use to guide decisions.

Collaborate with patients to form a treatment plan.

Monitor patients during use of dietary supplements.

full disclosure of use. Nonjudgmental questioning and demonstration of greater knowledge of the research concerning dietary supplements by physicians should aid in this endeavor. If the individual practitioner does not have this expertise, resources and referral sources should be identified to supplement their expertise.

Risks may be associated with the use of DS. These should be discussed specifically, based on evidence where possible (summary of evidence for risk or lack of harm is in Table 1). Caution should be urged when DS use substitutes for or delays the start of conventional care. Use of St. John's wort with chemotherapy and vitamin E in head and neck cancer patients should be discouraged. The use of blanket negative statements about DS to patients who perceive benefit from their use and have identified sources that support such use does not foster open communication.

Familiarity with the literature supporting safe dietary supplements, especially those used to relieve symptoms related to treatment, would help the clinician guide the patient toward supplements that are most likely to benefit them (summary of evidence for efficacy is in Table 2). A number of products reviewed here suggest benefit, including medicinal mushrooms and other immunomodulators, glutamine, ginger, black cohosh, and ω3FA, among others. Use of products that have been tested in clinical trials should be preferred where such products are available. Steering patients toward well-characterized products from reputable sources can address concerns regarding the quality of dietary supplements. Specific strategies to aid patients in deriving maximal benefit from their use of dietary supplements while minimizing risk are listed in Box 1. Finally, it is critical that further research on the combined use of DS and conventional cancer treatments be given higher priority. As our knowledge improves, so will our ability to advise our patients.

References

[1] D'Andrea GM. Use of antioxidants during chemotherapy and radiotherapy should be avoided. CA Cancer J Clin 2005;55(5):319–21.

[2] Yates JS, Mustian KM, Morrow GR, et al. Prevalence of complementary and alternative medicine use in cancer patients during treatment. Support Care Cancer 2005;13(10): 806–11.

[3] Molassiotis A, Ozden G, Platin N, et al. Complementary and alternative medicine use in patients with head and neck cancers in Europe. Eur J Cancer Care (Engl) 2006;15(1): 19–24.

[4] Vapiwala N, Mick R, Hampshire MK, Metz JM, DeNittis AS. Patient initiation of complementary and alternative medical therapies (CAM) following cancer diagnosis. Cancer J 2006;12(6):467–74.

[5] DiGianni LM, Kim HT, Emmons K, Gelman R, Kalkbrenner KJ, Garber JE. Complementary medicine use among women enrolled in a genetic testing program. Cancer Epidemiol Biomarkers Prev 2003;12(4):321–6.

[6] Digianni LM, Rue M, Emmons K, Garber JE. Complementary medicine use before and 1 year following genetic testing for BRCA1/2 mutations. Cancer Epidemiol Biomarkers Prev 2006;15(1):70–5.

[7] Gupta D, Lis CG, Birdsall TC, Grutsch JF. The use of dietary supplements in a community hospital comprehensive cancer center: implications for conventional cancer care. Support Care Cancer 2005;13(11):912–9.

[8] Sparber A, Bauer L, Curt G, et al. Use of complementary medicine by adult patients participating in cancer clinical trials. Oncol Nurs Forum 2000;27(4):623–30.

[9] Hlubocky FJ, Ratain MJ, Wen M, Daugherty CK. Complementary and alternative medicine among advanced cancer patients enrolled on phase I trials: a study of prognosis, quality of life, and preferences for decision making. J Clin Oncol 2007;25(5):548–54.

[10] Swarup AB, Barrett W, Jazieh AR. The use of complementary and alternative medicine by cancer patients undergoing radiation therapy. Am J Clin Oncol 2006;29(5):468–73.

[11] Hann D, Baker F, Denniston M, Entrekin N. Long-term breast cancer survivors' use of complementary therapies: perceived impact on recovery and prevention of recurrence. Integr Cancer Ther 2005;4(1):14–20.

[12] Jazieh AR, Kopp M, Foraida M, et al. The use of dietary supplements by veterans with cancer. J Altern Complement Med 2004;10(3):560–4.

[13] Tasaki K, Maskarinec G, Shumay DM, Tatsumura Y, Kakai H. Communication between physicians and cancer patients about complementary and alternative medicine: exploring patients' perspectives. Psychooncology 2002;11(3):212–20.

[14] Verhoef MJ, White MA, Doll R. Cancer patients' expectations of the role of family physicians in communication about complementary therapies. Cancer Prev Control 1999;3(3):181–7.

[15] Hyodo I, Eguchi K, Nishina T, et al. Perceptions and attitudes of clinical oncologists on complementary and alternative medicine: a nationwide survey in Japan. Cancer 2003;97(11):2861–8.

[16] Bourgeault IL. Physicians' attitudes toward patients' use of alternative cancer therapies. Cmaj 1996;155(12):1679–85.

[17] Richardson MA, Masse LC, Nanny K, Sanders C. Discrepant views of oncologists and cancer patients on complementary/alternative medicine. Support Care Cancer 2004;12(11): 797–804.

[18] Henderson JW, Donatelle RJ. Complementary and alternative medicine use by women after completion of allopathic treatment for breast cancer. Altern Ther Health Med 2004;10(1):52–7.

[19] Hann DM, Baker F, Roberts CS, et al. Use of complementary therapies among breast and prostate cancer patients during treatment: a multisite study. Integr Cancer Ther 2005;4(4): 294–300.

[20] Verhoef MJ, Mulkins A, Carlson LE, Hilsden RJ, Kania A. Assessing the role of evidence in patients' evaluation of complementary therapies: a quality study. Integr Cancer Ther 2007;6(4):345–53.

[21] Bauer B, Lee M, Wahner-Roedler D, Brown S, Pankratz S, Elkin PL. A controlled trial of physicians' amd patients' abilities to distinguish authoritative from misleading complementary and alternative medicine Web sites. Journal of Cancer Integrative Medicine 2003;1(1): 48–54.

[22] Ernst E, Cassileth BR. How useful are unconventional cancer treatments? Eur J Cancer 1999;35(11):1608–13.

[23] Chang EY, Glissmeyer M, Tonnes S, Hudson T, Johnson N. Outcomes of breast cancer in patients who use alternative therapies as primary treatment. Am J Surg 2006;192(4):471–3.

[24] Miller DR, Anderson GT, Stark JJ, Granick JL, Richardson D. Phase I/II trial of the safety and efficacy of shark cartilage in the treatment of advanced cancer. J Clin Oncol 1998;16(11): 3649–55.

[25] Loprinzi CL, Levitt R, Barton DL, et al. Evaluation of shark cartilage in patients with advanced cancer: a North Central Cancer Treatment Group trial. Cancer 2005;104(1): 176–82.

[26] Moertel CG, Fleming TR, Rubin J, et al. A clinical trial of amygdalin (Laetrile) in the treatment of human cancer. N Engl J Med 1982;306(4):201–6.

[27] Helyer LK, Chin S, Chui BK, et al. The use of complementary and alternative medicines among patients with locally advanced breast cancer–a descriptive study. BMC Cancer 2006;6:39.

[28] Cassileth BR, Lusk EJ, Strouse TB, Bodenheimer BJ. Contemporary unorthodox treatments in cancer medicine. A study of patients, treatments, and practitioners. Ann Intern Med 1984;101(1):105–12.

[29] Cassileth BR, Lusk EJ, Guerry D, et al. Survival and quality of life among patients receiving unproven as compared with conventional cancer therapy. N Engl J Med 1991;324(17): 1180–5.

[30] Cosyns JP. Aristolochic acid and "Chinese herbs nephropathy": a review of the evidence to date. Drug Saf 2003;26(1):33–48.

[31] White J. PC-SPES–a lesson for future dietary supplement research. J Natl Cancer Inst 2002;94(17):1261–3.

[32] Guns ES, Goldenberg SL, Brown PN. Mass spectral analysis of PC-SPES confirms the presence of diethylstilbestrol. Can J Urol 2002;9(6):1684–8, discussion 1689.

[33] Fact Sheet Dietary Supplement Current Good Manufacturing Practices (CGMPs) and Interim Final Rule (IFR) Facts. Available at: http://www.cfsan.fda.gov/~dms/dscgmps6.html.

[34] McGuffin M, Hobbs C, Upton R, Goldberg A, editors. American Herbal Product Association's Botanical Safety Handbook. Boca Raton, Florida: CRC Press; 1997. p. 129–60.

[35] Seeff LB. Herbal hepatotoxicity. Clin Liver Dis 2007;11(3):577–96, vii.

[36] Blumenthal M. European Health Agencies Recommend Liver Warnings on Black Cohosh Products. Herbalgram 2006;72:56–8.

[37] Report on Workshop on the Safety of Black Cohosh in Clinical Studies. Paper presented at: Workshop on the Safety of Black Cohosh in Clinical Studies, 2004; National Institutes of Health Bethesda, Maryland. Available at: http://nccam.nih.gov/news/pastmeetings/blackcohosh_mtngsumm.html.

[38] Sparreboom A, Cox MC, Acharya MR, Figg WD. Herbal remedies in the United States: potential adverse interactions with anticancer agents. J Clin Oncol 2004;22(12): 2489–503.

[39] Yeung KS, Gubili J. Clinical guide to herb-drug interactions in oncology. J Soc Integr Oncol 2007;5(3):113–7.

[40] Meijerman I, Beijnen JH, Schellens JH. Herb-drug interactions in oncology: focus on mechanisms of induction. Oncologist 2006;11(7):742–52.

[41] McCune JS, Hatfield AJ, Blackburn AA, Leith PO, Livingston RB, Ellis GK. Potential of chemotherapy-herb interactions in adult cancer patients. Support Care Cancer 2004;12(6): 454–62.

[42] Block KI, Gyllenhaal C. Clinical corner: herb-drug interactions in cancer chemotherapy: theoretical concerns regarding drug metabolizing enzymes. Integr Cancer Ther 2002;1(1):83–9.

[43] Werneke U, Earl J, Seydel C, Horn O, Crichton P, Fannon D. Potential health risks of complementary alternative medicines in cancer patients. Br J Cancer 2004;90(2):408–13.

[44] Skalli S, Zaid A, Soulaymani R. Drug interactions with herbal medicines. Ther Drug Monit 2007;29(6):679–86.

[45] Cox MC, Low J, Lee J, et al. Influence of garlic (Allium sativum) on the pharmacokinetics of docetaxel. Clin Cancer Res 2006;12(15):4636–40.

[46] van Erp NP, Baker SD, Zhao M, et al. Effect of milk thistle (Silybum marianum) on the pharmacokinetics of irinotecan. Clin Cancer Res 2005;11(21):7800–6.

[47] Smith P, Bullock JM, Booker BM, Haas CE, Berenson CS, Jusko WJ. The influence of St. John's wort on the pharmacokinetics and protein binding of imatinib mesylate. Pharmacotherapy 2004;24(11):1508–14.

[48] Frye RF, Fitzgerald SM, Lagattuta TF, Hruska MW, Egorin MJ. Effect of St John's wort on imatinib mesylate pharmacokinetics. Clin Pharmacol Ther 2004;76(4):323–9.

[49] Mathijssen RH, Verweij J, de Bruijn P, Loos WJ, Sparreboom A. Effects of St. John's wort on irinotecan metabolism. J Natl Cancer Inst 2002;94(16):1247–9.

[50] Mannel M. Drug interactions with St John's wort: mechanisms and clinical implications. Drug Saf 2004;27(11):773–97.

[51] Kumar NB, Allen K, Bell H. Perioperative herbal supplement use in cancer patients: potential implications and recommendations for presurgical screening. Cancer Control 2005;12(3):149–57.

[52] Beckert BW, Concannon MJ, Henry SL, Smith DS, Puckett CL. The effect of herbal medicines on platelet function: an in vivo experiment and review of the literature. Plast Reconstr Surg 2007;120(7):2044–50.

[53] Wittkowsky AK. Dietary supplements, herbs and oral anticoagulants: the nature of the evidence. J Thromb Thrombolysis 2008;25(1):72–7.

[54] Piersen CE. Phytoestrogens in botanical dietary supplements: implications for cancer. Integr Cancer Ther 2003;2(2):120–38.

[55] Beck V, Unterrieder E, Krenn L, Kubelka W, Jungbauer A. Comparison of hormonal activity (estrogen, androgen and progestin) of standardized plant extracts for large scale use in hormone replacement therapy. J Steroid Biochem Mol Biol 2003;84(2–3):259–68.

[56] Lupu R, Mehmi I, Atlas E, et al. Black cohosh, a menopausal remedy, does not have estrogenic activity and does not promote breast cancer cell growth. Int J Oncol 2003;23(5):1407–12.

[57] Walji R, Boon H, Guns E, Oneschuk D, Younus J. Black cohosh (Cimicifuga racemosa [L.] Nutt.): safety and efficacy for cancer patients. Support Care Cancer 2007;15(8):913–21.

[58] Raus K, Brucker C, Gorkow C, Wuttke W. First-time proof of endometrial safety of the special black cohosh extract (Actaea or Cimicifuga racemosa extract) CR BNO 1055. Menopause 2006;13(4):678–91.

[59] Hirschberg AL, Edlund M, Svane G, Azavedo E, Skoog L, von Schoultz B. An isopropanolic extract of black cohosh does not increase mammographic breast density or breast cell proliferation in postmenopausal women. Menopause 2007;14(1):89–96.

[60] Burdette JE, Liu J, Chen SN, et al. Black cohosh acts as a mixed competitive ligand and partial agonist of the serotonin receptor. J Agric Food Chem 2003;51(19):5661–70.

[61] Shekelle P, Hardy ML, Coulter I, et al. Effect of the supplemental use of antioxidants vitamin C, vitamin E, and coenzyme Q10 for the prevention and treatment of cancer. Evid Rep Technol Assess (Summ) 2003;75:1–3.

[62] Omenn GS. Chemoprevention of lung cancers: lessons from CARET, the beta-carotene and retinol efficacy trial, and prospects for the future. Eur J Cancer Prev 2007;16(3):184–91.

[63] Prasad KN, Cole WC, Kumar B, Prasad KC. Scientific rationale for using high-dose multiple micronutrients as an adjunct to standard and experimental cancer therapies. J Am Coll Nutr 2001;20(5 Suppl):450S–63S; discussion 473S–5S.

[64] Moss RW. Should patients undergoing chemotherapy and radiotherapy be prescribed antioxidants? Integr Cancer Ther 2006;5(1):63–82.

[65] Simone CB 2nd, Simone NL, Simone V, Simone CB. Antioxidants and other nutrients do not interfere with chemotherapy or radiation therapy and can increase kill and increase survival, Part 2. Altern Ther Health Med 2007;13(2):40–7.

[66] Simone CB 2nd, Simone NL, Simone V, Simone CB. Antioxidants and other nutrients do not interfere with chemotherapy or radiation therapy and can increase kill and increase survival, part 1. Altern Ther Health Med 2007;13(1):22–8.

[67] Prasad KN. Rationale for using multiple antioxidants in protecting humans against low doses of ionizing radiation. Br J Radiol 2005;78(930):485–92.

[68] Bairati I, Meyer F, Gelinas M, et al. Randomized trial of antioxidant vitamins to prevent acute adverse effects of radiation therapy in head and neck cancer patients. J Clin Oncol 2005;23(24):5805–13.

[69] Bairati I, Meyer F, Jobin E, et al. Antioxidant vitamins supplementation and mortality: a randomized trial in head and neck cancer patients. Int J Cancer 2006;119(9):2221–4.

[70] Lesperance ML, Olivotto IA, Forde N, et al. Mega-dose vitamins and minerals in the treatment of non-metastatic breast cancer: an historical cohort study. Breast Cancer Res Treat 2002;76(2):137–43.

[71] Pathak AK, Bhutani M, Guleria R, et al. Chemotherapy alone vs. chemotherapy plus high dose multiple antioxidants in patients with advanced non small cell lung cancer. J Am Coll Nutr 2005;24(1):16–21.

[72] Cameron E, Pauling L. Supplemental ascorbate in the supportive treatment of cancer: reevaluation of prolongation of survival times in terminal human cancer. Proc Natl Acad Sci U S A 1978;75(9):4538–42.

[73] Moertel CG, Fleming TR, Creagan ET, Rubin J, O'Connell MJ, Ames MM. High-dose vitamin C versus placebo in the treatment of patients with advanced cancer who have had no prior chemotherapy. A randomized double-blind comparison. N Engl J Med 1985;312(3):137–41.

[74] Creagan ET, Moertel CG, O'Fallon JR, et al. Failure of high-dose vitamin C (ascorbic acid) therapy to benefit patients with advanced cancer. A controlled trial. N Engl J Med 1979;301(13):687–90.

[75] Drisko JA, Chapman J, Hunter VJ. The use of antioxidants with first-line chemotherapy in two cases of ovarian cancer. J Am Coll Nutr 2003;22(2):118–23.

[76] Drisko JA, Chapman J, Hunter VJ. The use of antioxidant therapies during chemotherapy. Gynecol Oncol 2003;88(3):434–9.

[77] Kennedy DD, Tucker KL, Ladas ED, Rheingold SR, Blumberg J, Kelly KM. Low antioxidant vitamin intakes are associated with increases in adverse effects of chemotherapy in children with acute lymphoblastic leukemia. Am J Clin Nutr 2004;79(6):1029–36.

[78] Weijl NI, Elsendoorn TJ, Lentjes EG, et al. Supplementation with antioxidant micronutrients and chemotherapy-induced toxicity in cancer patients treated with cisplatin-based chemotherapy: a randomised, double-blind, placebo-controlled study. Eur J Cancer 2004;40(11):1713–23.

[79] Conklin KA. Coenzyme q10 for prevention of anthracycline-induced cardiotoxicity. Integr Cancer Ther 2005;4(2):110–30.

[80] Strasser F, Luftner D, Possinger K, et al. Comparison of orally administered cannabis extract and delta-9-tetrahydrocannabinol in treating patients with cancer-related anorexia-cachexia syndrome: a multicenter, phase III, randomized, double-blind, placebo-controlled clinical trial from the Cannabis-In-Cachexia-Study-Group. J Clin Oncol 2006;24(21):3394–400.

[81] Kidd PM. The use of mushroom glucans and proteoglycans in cancer treatment. Altern Med Rev 2000;5(1):4–27.

[82] Wasser SP. Medicinal mushrooms as a source of antitumor and immunomodulating poly-saccharides. Appl Microbiol Biotechnol 2002;60(3):258–74.

[83] Borchers AT, Stern JS, Hackman RM, Keen CL, Gershwin ME. Mushrooms, tumors, and immunity. Proc Soc Exp Biol Med 1999;221(4):281–93.

[84] Akramiene D, Kondrotas A, Didziapetriene J, Kevelaitis E. Effects of beta-glucans on the immune system. Medicina (Kaunas) 2007;43(8):597–606.

[85] Ohwada S, Ogawa T, Makita F, et al. Beneficial effects of protein-bound polysaccharide K plus tegafur/uracil in patients with stage II or III colorectal cancer: analysis of immunological parameters. Oncol Rep 2006;15(4):861–8.

[86] Ohwada S, Ikeya T, Yokomori T, et al. Adjuvant immunochemotherapy with oral Tegafur/Uracil plus PSK in patients with stage II or III colorectal cancer: a randomised controlled study. Br J Cancer 2004;90(5):1003–10.

[87] Sakamoto J, Morita S, Oba K, et al. Efficacy of adjuvant immunochemotherapy with polysaccharide K for patients with curatively resected colorectal cancer: a meta-analysis of centrally randomized controlled clinical trials. Cancer Immunol Immunother 2006;55(4):404–11.

[88] Oba K, Teramukai S, Kobayashi M, Matsui T, Kodera Y, Sakamoto J. Efficacy of adjuvant immunochemotherapy with polysaccharide K for patients with curative resections of gastric cancer. Cancer Immunol Immunother 2007;56(6):905–11.

[89] Nakazato H, Koike A, Saji S, Ogawa N, Sakamoto J. Efficacy of immunochemotherapy as adjuvant treatment after curative resection of gastric cancer. Study Group of Immunochemotherapy with PSK for Gastric Cancer. Lancet 1994;343(8906):1122–6.

[90] Bao YX, Wong CK, Leung SF, et al. Clinical studies of immunomodulatory activities of Yunzhi-Danshen in patients with nasopharyngeal carcinoma. J Altern Complement Med 2006;12(8):771–6.

[91] Wong CK, Bao YX, Wong EL, Leung PC, Fung KP, Lam CW. Immunomodulatory activities of Yunzhi and Danshen in post-treatment breast cancer patients. Am J Chin Med 2005;33(3):381–95.

[92] Ghoneum M, Wimbley M, Salem F, McKlain A, ATtallah N, Gill G. Immunomodulatory and Anticancer effects of Active Hemicellulose Compound (AHCC). International Journal of Immunotherapy 1995;11(1):23–8.

[93] Cowawintaweewat S, Manoromana S, Sriplung H, et al. Prognostic improvement of patients with advanced liver cancer after active hexose correlated compound (AHCC) treatment. Asian Pac J Allergy Immunol 2006;24(1):33–45.

[94] Matsui Y, Uhara J, Satoi S, et al. Improved prognosis of postoperative hepatocellular carcinoma patients when treated with functional foods: a prospective cohort study. J Hepatol 2002;37(1):78–86.

[95] Yang D, Li S, Wang H, et al. [Prevention of postoperative recurrence of bladder cancer: a clinical study]. Zhonghua Wai Ke Za Zhi 1999;37(8):464–5 [in Chinese].

[96] Kodama N, Komuta K, Nanba H. Effect of Maitake (Grifola frondosa) D-Fraction on the activation of NK cells in cancer patients. J Med Food 2003;6(4):371–7.

[97] Chen X, Hu ZP, Yang XX, et al. Monitoring of immune responses to a herbal immuno-modulator in patients with advanced colorectal cancer. Int Immunopharmacol 2006;6(3):499–508.

[98] Gao Y, Zhou S, Jiang W, Huang M, Dai X. Effects of ganopoly (a Ganoderma lucidum polysaccharide extract) on the immune functions in advanced-stage cancer patients. Immunol Invest 2003;32(3):201–15.

[99] Gao Y, Tang W, Dai X, et al. Effects of water-soluble Ganoderma lucidum polysaccharides on the immune functions of patients with advanced lung cancer. J Med Food 2005;8(2):159–68.

[100] Ahn WS, Kim DJ, Chae GT, et al. Natural killer cell activity and quality of life were improved by consumption of a mushroom extract, Agaricus blazei Murill Kyowa, in gynecological cancer patients undergoing chemotherapy. Int J Gynecol Cancer 2004;14(4):589–94.

[101] Boros LG, Nichelatti M, Shoenfeld Y. Fermented wheat germ extract (Avemar) in the treatment of cancer and autoimmune diseases. Ann N Y Acad Sci 2005;1051:529–42.

[102] Garami M, Schuler D, Babosa M, et al. Fermented wheat germ extract reduces chemotherapy-induced febrile neutropenia in pediatric cancer patients. J Pediatr Hematol Oncol 2004;26(10):631–5.

[103] Jakab F, Shoenfeld Y, Balogh A, et al. A medical nutriment has supportive value in the treatment of colorectal cancer. Br J Cancer 2003;89(3):465–9.

[104] Demidov L, Manzjuk L, Kharkevitch G, Artamonova E, Pirogova N. Antimetastatic effect of Avemar in high-risk melanoma patietns. 18th UICC International Cancer Congress. Oslo: Norway; 2002.

[105] Mego M, Koncekova R, Mikuskova E, et al. Prevention of febrile neutropenia in cancer patients by probiotic strain Enterococcus faecium M-74. Phase II study. Support Care Cancer 2006;14(3):285–90.

[106] Sugawara G, Nagino M, Nishio H, et al. Perioperative synbiotic treatment to prevent postoperative infectious complications in biliary cancer surgery: a randomized controlled trial. Ann Surg 2006;244(5):706–14.

[107] Besselink MG, van Santvoort HC, Buskens E, et al. Probiotic prophylaxis in predicted severe acute pancreatitis: a randomised, double-blind, placebo-controlled trial. Lancet 2008;371(9613):651–9.

[108] Alterio D, Jereczek-Fossa BA, Fiore MR, Piperno G, Ansarin M, Orecchia R. Cancer treatment-induced oral mucositis. Anticancer Res 2007;27(2):1105–25.

[109] Kaul R, Mishra BK, Sutradar P, Choudhary V, Gujral MS. The role of Wobe-Mugos in reducing acute sequele of radiation in head and neck cancers–a clinical phase-III randomized trial. Indian J Cancer 1999;36(2–4):141–8.

[110] Nikoletti S, Hyde S, Shaw T, Myers H, Kristjanson LJ. Comparison of plain ice and flavoured ice for preventing oral mucositis associated with the use of 5 fluorouracil. J Clin Nurs 2005;14(6):750–3.

[111] Biswal BM, Zakaria A, Ahmad NM. Topical application of honey in the management of radiation mucositis: a preliminary study. Support Care Cancer 2003;11(4):242–8.

[112] Cerchietti LC, Navigante AH, Lutteral MA, et al. Double-blinded, placebo-controlled trial on intravenous L-alanyl-L-glutamine in the incidence of oral mucositis following chemoradiotherapy in patients with head-and-neck cancer. Int J Radiat Oncol Biol Phys 2006;65(5):1330–7.

[113] Rubio IT, Cao Y, Hutchins LF, Westbrook KC, Klimberg VS. Effect of glutamine on methotrexate efficacy and toxicity. Ann Surg 1998;227(5):772–8, discussion 778–80.

[114] Anderson PM, Schroeder G, Skubitz KM. Oral glutamine reduces the duration and severity of stomatitis after cytotoxic cancer chemotherapy. Cancer 1998;83(7):1433–9.

[115] Skubitz KM, Anderson PM. Oral glutamine to prevent chemotherapy induced stomatitis: a pilot study. J Lab Clin Med 1996;127(2):223–8.

[116] Anderson PM, Ramsay NK, Shu XO, et al. Effect of low-dose oral glutamine on painful stomatitis during bone marrow transplantation. Bone Marrow Transplant 1998;22(4):339–44.

[117] Aquino VM, Harvey AR, Garvin JH, et al. A double-blind randomized placebo-controlled study of oral glutamine in the prevention of mucositis in children undergoing hematopoietic stem cell transplantation: a pediatric blood and marrow transplant consortium study. Bone Marrow Transplant 2005;36(7):611–6.

[118] Cockerham MB, Weinberger BB, Lerchie SB. Oral glutamine for the prevention of oral mucositis associated with high-dose paclitaxel and melphalan for autologous bone marrow transplantation. Ann Pharmacother 2000;34(3):300–3.

[119] Huang EY, Leung SW, Wang CJ, et al. Oral glutamine to alleviate radiation-induced oral mucositis: a pilot randomized trial. Int J Radiat Oncol Biol Phys 2000;46(3):535–9.

[120] Okuno SH, Woodhouse CO, Loprinzi CL, et al. Phase III controlled evaluation of glutamine for decreasing stomatitis in patients receiving fluorouracil (5-FU)-based chemotherapy. Am J Clin Oncol 1999;22(3):258–61.

[121] Jebb SA, Osborne RJ, Maughan TS, et al. 5-fluorouracil and folinic acid-induced mucositis: no effect of oral glutamine supplementation. Br J Cancer 1994;70(4):732–5.

[122] El-Housseiny AA, Saleh SM, El-Masry AA, Allam AA. The effectiveness of vitamin "E" in the treatment of oral mucositis in children receiving chemotherapy. J Clin Pediatr Dent 2007;31(3):167–70.

[123] Sung L, Tomlinson GA, Greenberg ML, et al. Serial controlled N-of-1 trials of topical vitamin E as prophylaxis for chemotherapy-induced oral mucositis in paediatric patients. Eur J Cancer 2007;43(8):1269–75.

[124] Wadleigh RG, Redman RS, Graham ML, Krasnow SH, Anderson A, Cohen MH. Vitamin E in the treatment of chemotherapy-induced mucositis. Am J Med 1992;92(5):481–4.

[125] Ferreira PR, Fleck JF, Diehl A, et al. Protective effect of alpha-tocopherol in head and neck cancer radiation-induced mucositis: a double-blind randomized trial. Head Neck 2004;26(4):313–21.

[126] Lin LC, Que J, Lin LK, Lin FC. Zinc supplementation to improve mucositis and dermatitis in patients after radiotherapy for head-and-neck cancers: a double-blind, randomized study. Int J Radiat Oncol Biol Phys 2006;65(3):745–50.

[127] Ertekin MV, Koc M, Karslioglu I, Sezen O. Zinc sulfate in the prevention of radiation-induced oropharyngeal mucositis: a prospective, placebo-controlled, randomized study. Int J Radiat Oncol Biol Phys 2004;58(1):167–74.

[128] Su CK, Mehta V, Ravikumar L, et al. Phase II double-blind randomized study comparing oral aloe vera versus placebo to prevent radiation-related mucositis in patients with head-and-neck neoplasms. Int J Radiat Oncol Biol Phys 2004;60(1):171–7.

[129] Carl W, Emrich LS. Management of oral mucositis during local radiation and systemic chemotherapy: a study of 98 patients. J Prosthet Dent 1991;66(3):361–9.

[130] Mazokopakis EE, Vrentzos GE, Papadakis JA, Babalis DE, Ganotakis ES. Wild chamomile (Matricaria recutita L.) mouthwashes in methotrexate-induced oral mucositis. Phytomedicine 2005;12(1–2):25–7.

[131] Fidler P, Loprinzi CL, O'Fallon JR, et al. Prospective evaluation of a chamomile mouthwash for prevention of 5-FU-induced oral mucositis. Cancer 1996;77(3):522–5.

[132] Oberbaum M, Yaniv I, Ben-Gal Y, et al. A randomized, controlled clinical trial of the homeopathic medication TRAUMEEL S in the treatment of chemotherapy-induced stomatitis in children undergoing stem cell transplantation. Cancer 2001;92(3):684–90.

[133] Gujral MS, Patnaik PM, Kaul R, et al. Efficacy of hydrolytic enzymes in preventing radiation therapy-induced side effects in patients with head and neck cancers. Cancer Chemother Pharmacol 2001;47(Suppl):S23–28.

[134] Melichar B, Kohout P, Bratova M, Solichova D, Kralickova P, Zadak Z. Intestinal permeability in patients with chemotherapy-induced stomatitis. J Cancer Res Clin Oncol 2001;127(5):314–8.

[135] Choi K, Lee SS, Oh SJ, et al. The effect of oral glutamine on 5-fluorouracil/leucovorin-induced mucositis/stomatitis assessed by intestinal permeability test. Clin Nutr 2007;26(1):57–62.

[136] Osterlund P, Ruotsalainen T, Peuhkuri K, et al. Lactose intolerance associated with adjuvant 5-fluorouracil-based chemotherapy for colorectal cancer. Clin Gastroenterol Hepatol 2004;2(8):696–703.

[137] Savarese DM, Savy G, Vahdat L, Wischmeyer PE, Corey B. Prevention of chemotherapy and radiation toxicity with glutamine. Cancer Treat Rev 2003;29(6):501–13.

[138] Daniele B, Perrone F, Gallo C, et al. Oral glutamine in the prevention of fluorouracil induced intestinal toxicity: a double blind, placebo controlled, randomised trial. Gut 2001;48(1):28–33.

[139] Savarese D, Al-Zoubi A, Boucher J. Glutamine for irinotecan diarrhea. J Clin Oncol 2000;18(2):450–1.

[140] Li Y, Yu Z, Liu F, Tan L, Wu B, Li J. Oral glutamine ameliorates chemotherapy-induced changes of intestinal permeability and does not interfere with the antitumor effect of

chemotherapy in patients with breast cancer: a prospective randomized trial. Tumori 2006;92(5):396–401.

[141] Bozzetti F, Biganzoli L, Gavazzi C, et al. Glutamine supplementation in cancer patients receiving chemotherapy: a double-blind randomized study. Nutrition 1997;13(7-8):748–51.

[142] Kozelsky TF, Meyers GE, Sloan JA, et al. Phase III double-blind study of glutamine versus placebo for the prevention of acute diarrhea in patients receiving pelvic radiation therapy. J Clin Oncol 2003;21(9):1669–74.

[143] Osterlund P, Ruotsalainen T, Korpela R, et al. Lactobacillus supplementation for diarrhoea related to chemotherapy of colorectal cancer: a randomised study. Br J Cancer 2007;97(8):1028–34.

[144] Urbancsek H, Kazar T, Mezes I, Neumann K. Results of a double-blind, randomized study to evaluate the efficacy and safety of Antibiophilus in patients with radiation-induced diarrhoea. Eur J Gastroenterol Hepatol 2001;13(4):391–6.

[145] Delia P, Sansotta G, Donato V, et al. Prevention of radiation-induced diarrhea with the use of VSL#3, a new high-potency probiotic preparation. Am J Gastroenterol 2002;97(8):2150–2.

[146] Delia P, Sansotta G, Donato V, et al. Use of probiotics for prevention of radiation-induced diarrhea. World J Gastroenterol 2007;13(6):912–5.

[147] Stillman M, Cata JP. Management of chemotherapy-induced peripheral neuropathy. Curr Pain Headache Rep 2006;10(4):279–87.

[148] Vahdat L, Papadopoulos K, Lange D, et al. Reduction of paclitaxel-induced peripheral neuropathy with glutamine. Clin Cancer Res 2001;7(5):1192–7.

[149] Stubblefield MD, Vahdat LT, Balmaceda CM, Troxel AB, Hesdorffer CS, Gooch CL. Glutamine as a neuroprotective agent in high-dose paclitaxel-induced peripheral neuropathy: a clinical and electrophysiologic study. Clin Oncol (R Coll Radiol) 2005;17(4):271–6.

[150] Wang WS, Lin JK, Lin TC, et al. Oral glutamine is effective for preventing oxaliplatin-induced neuropathy in colorectal cancer patients. Oncologist 2007;12(3):312–9.

[151] Pace A, Savarese A, Picardo M, et al. Neuroprotective effect of vitamin E supplementation in patients treated with cisplatin chemotherapy. J Clin Oncol 2003;21(5):927–31.

[152] Argyriou AA, Chroni E, Koutras A, et al. Vitamin E for prophylaxis against chemotherapy-induced neuropathy: a randomized controlled trial. Neurology 2005;64(1):26–31.

[153] Argyriou AA, Chroni E, Koutras A, et al. Preventing paclitaxel-induced peripheral neuropathy: a phase II trial of vitamin E supplementation. J Pain Symptom Manage 2006;32(3): 237–44.

[154] Argyriou AA, Chroni E, Koutras A, et al. A randomized controlled trial evaluating the efficacy and safety of vitamin E supplementation for protection against cisplatin-induced peripheral neuropathy: final results. Support Care Cancer 2006;14(11):1134–40.

[155] Nanthakomon T, Pongrojpaw D. The efficacy of ginger in prevention of postoperative nausea and vomiting after major gynecologic surgery. J Med Assoc Thai 2006;89(Suppl 4): S130–6.

[156] Meyer K, Schwartz J, Crater D, Keyes B. Zingiber officinale (ginger) used to prevent 8-Mop associated nausea. Dermatol Nurs 1995;7(4):242–4.

[157] Manusirivithaya S, Sripramote M, Tangjitgamol S, et al. Antiemetic effect of ginger in gynecologic oncology patients receiving cisplatin. Int J Gynecol Cancer 2004;14(6): 1063–9.

[158] Richardson J, Smith JE, McIntyre M, Thomas R, Pilkington K. Aloe vera for preventing radiation-induced skin reactions: a systematic literature review. Clin Oncol (R Coll Radiol) 2005;17(6):478–84.

[159] Olsen DL, Raub W Jr, Bradley C, et al. The effect of aloe vera gel/mild soap versus mild soap alone in preventing skin reactions in patients undergoing radiation therapy. Oncol Nurs Forum 2001;28(3):543–7.

[160] Williams MS, Burk M, Loprinzi CL, et al. Phase III double-blind evaluation of an aloe vera gel as a prophylactic agent for radiation-induced skin toxicity. Int J Radiat Oncol Biol Phys 1996;36(2):345–9.

[161] Maiche AG, Grohn P, Maki-Hokkonen H. Effect of chamomile cream and almond ointment on acute radiation skin reaction. Acta Oncol 1991;30(3):395–6.

[162] Pommier P, Gomez F, Sunyach MP, D'Hombres A, Carrie C, Montbarbon X. Phase III randomized trial of Calendula officinalis compared with trolamine for the prevention of acute dermatitis during irradiation for breast cancer. J Clin Oncol 2004;22(8):1447–53.

[163] Dewey A, Baughan C, Dean T, Higgins B, Johnson I. Eicosapentaenoic acid (EPA, an omega-3 fatty acid from fish oils) for the treatment of cancer cachexia. Cochrane Database Syst Rev 2007;(1):CD004597.

[164] Colomer R, Moreno-Nogueira JM, Garcia-Luna PP, et al. N-3 fatty acids, cancer and cachexia: a systematic review of the literature. Br J Nutr 2007;97(5):823–31.

[165] Elia M, Van Bokhorst-de van der Schueren MA, Garvey J, et al. Enteral (oral or tube administration) nutritional support and eicosapentaenoic acid in patients with cancer: a systematic review. Int J Oncol 2006;28(1):5–23.

[166] Burns CP, Halabi S, Clamon GH, et al. Phase I clinical study of fish oil fatty acid capsules for patients with cancer cachexia: cancer and leukemia group B study 9473. Clin Cancer Res 1999;5(12):3942–7.

[167] Cerchietti LC, Navigante AH, Castro MA. Effects of eicosapentaenoic and docosahexaenoic n-3 fatty acids from fish oil and preferential Cox-2 inhibition on systemic syndromes in patients with advanced lung cancer. Nutr Cancer 2007;59(1):14–20.

[168] Burns CP, Halabi S, Clamon G, et al. Phase II study of high-dose fish oil capsules for patients with cancer-related cachexia. Cancer 2004;101(2):370–8.

[169] Jatoi A, Rowland K, Loprinzi CL, et al. An eicosapentaenoic acid supplement versus megestrol acetate versus both for patients with cancer-associated wasting: a North Central Cancer Treatment Group and National Cancer Institute of Canada collaborative effort. J Clin Oncol 2004;22(12):2469–76.

[170] Mantovani G, Maccio A, Madeddu C, et al. A phase II study with antioxidants, both in the diet and supplemented, pharmaconutritional support, progestagen, and anti-cyclooxygenase-2 showing efficacy and safety in patients with cancer-related anorexia/cachexia and oxidative stress. Cancer Epidemiol Biomarkers Prev 2006;15(5):1030–4.

[171] Gothard L, Cornes P, Earl J, et al. Double-blind placebo-controlled randomised trial of vitamin E and pentoxifylline in patients with chronic arm lymphoedema and fibrosis after surgery and radiotherapy for breast cancer. Radiother Oncol 2004;73(2):133–9.

[172] Kasseroller RG, Schrauzer GN. Treatment of secondary lymphedema of the arm with physical decongestive therapy and sodium selenite: a review. Am J Ther 2000;7(4):273–9.

[173] Micke O, Bruns F, Mucke R, et al. Selenium in the treatment of radiation-associated secondary lymphedema. Int J Radiat Oncol Biol Phys 2003;56(1):40–9.

[174] Cluzan RV, Pecking AP, Mathiex-Fortunet H, Leger Picherit E. Efficacy of BN165 (Ginkor Fort) in breast cancer related upper limb lymphedema: a preliminary study. Lymphology 2004;37(2):47–52.

[175] Pecking AP. Evaluation by lymphoscintigraphy of the effect of a micronized flavonoid fraction (Daflon 500 mg) in the treatment of upper limb lymphedema. Int Angiol 1995;14(3 Suppl 1):39–43.

[176] Pecking AP, Fevrier B, Wargon C, Pillion G. Efficacy of Daflon 500 mg in the treatment of lymphedema (secondary to conventional therapy of breast cancer). Angiology 1997;48(1):93–8.

[177] Olszewski W. Clinical efficacy of micronized purified flavonoid fraction (MPFF) in edema. Angiology 2000;51(1):25–9.

[178] Cluzan RV, Alliot F, Ghabboun S, Pascot M. Treatment of secondary lymphedema of the upper limb with CYCLO 3 FORT. Lymphology 1996;29(1):29–35.

[179] Brooker S, Martin S, Pearson A, et al. Double-blind, placebo-controlled, randomised phase II trial of IH636 grape seed proanthocyanidin extract (GSPE) in patients with radiation-induced breast induration. Radiother Oncol 2006;79(1):45–51.

[180] Bruns F, Micke O, Bremer M. Current status of selenium and other treatments for secondary lymphedema. J Support Oncol 2003;1(2):121–30.

[181] Bruns F, Buntzel J, Mucke R, Schonekaes K, Kisters K, Micke O. Selenium in the treatment of head and neck lymphedema. Med Princ Pract 2004;13(4):185–90.

[182] Zimmermann T, Leonhardt H, Kersting S, Albrecht S, Range U, Eckelt U. Reduction of post-operative lymphedema after oral tumor surgery with sodium selenite. Biol Trace Elem Res 2005;106(3):193–203.

[183] de Souza Fede AB, Bensi CG, Trufelli DC, et al. Multivitamins do not improve radiation therapy-related fatigue: results of a double-blind randomized crossover trial. Am J Clin Oncol 2007;30(4):432–6.

[184] Cruciani RA, Dvorkin E, Homel P, et al. L-carnitine supplementation for the treatment of fatigue and depressed mood in cancer patients with carnitine deficiency: a preliminary analysis. Ann N Y Acad Sci 2004;1033:168–76.

[185] Graziano F, Bisonni R, Catalano V, et al. Potential role of levocarnitine supplementation for the treatment of chemotherapy-induced fatigue in non-anaemic cancer patients. Br J Cancer 2002;86(12):1854–7.

[186] Gramignano G, Lusso MR, Madeddu C, et al. Efficacy of l-carnitine administration on fatigue, nutritional status, oxidative stress, and related quality of life in 12 advanced cancer patients undergoing anticancer therapy. Nutrition 2006;22(2):136–45.

[187] Cruciani RA, Dvorkin E, Homel P, et al. Safety, tolerability and symptom outcomes associated with L-carnitine supplementation in patients with cancer, fatigue, and carnitine deficiency: a phase I/II study. J Pain Symptom Manage 2006;32(6):551–9.

[188] Jacobson JS, Troxel AB, Evans J, et al. Randomized trial of black cohosh for the treatment of hot flashes among women with a history of breast cancer. J Clin Oncol 2001;19(10): 2739–45.

[189] Pockaj BA, Loprinzi CL, Sloan JA, et al. Pilot evaluation of black cohosh for the treatment of hot flashes in women. Cancer Invest 2004;22(4):515–21.

[190] Pockaj BA, Gallagher JG, Loprinzi CL, et al. Phase III double-blind, randomized, placebo-controlled crossover trial of black cohosh in the management of hot flashes: NCCTG Trial N01CC1. J Clin Oncol 2006;24(18):2836–41.

[191] Hernandez Munoz G, Pluchino S. Cimicifuga racemosa for the treatment of hot flushes in women surviving breast cancer. Maturitas 2003;44(Suppl 1):S59–65.

[192] Rebbeck TR, Troxel AB, Norman S, et al. A retrospective case-control study of the use of hormone-related supplements and association with breast cancer. Int J Cancer 2007;120(7):1523–8.

[193] Zepelin HH, Meden H, Kostev K, Schroder-Bernhardi D, Stammwitz U, Becher H. Isopropanolic black cohosh extract and recurrence-free survival after breast cancer. Int J Clin Pharmacol Ther 2007;45(3):143–54.

[194] Li N, Sun Z, Han C, Chen J. The chemopreventive effects of tea on human oral precancerous mucosa lesions. Proc Soc Exp Biol Med 1999;220(4):218–24.

[195] Halder A, Raychowdhury R, Ghosh A, De M. Black tea (Camellia sinensis) as a chemopreventive agent in oral precancerous lesions. J Environ Pathol Toxicol Oncol 2005;24(2): 141–4.

[196] Bettuzzi S, Brausi M, Rizzi F, Castagnetti G, Peracchia G, Corti A. Chemoprevention of human prostate cancer by oral administration of green tea catechins in volunteers with high-grade prostate intraepithelial neoplasia: a preliminary report from a one-year proof-of-principle study. Cancer Res 2006;66(2):1234–40.

[197] Pantuck AJ, Leppert JT, Zomorodian N, et al. Phase II study of pomegranate juice for men with rising prostate-specific antigen following surgery or radiation for prostate cancer. Clin Cancer Res 2006;12(13):4018–26.

[198] Schroder FH, Roobol MJ, Boeve ER, et al. Randomized, double-blind, placebo-controlled crossover study in men with prostate cancer and rising PSA: effectiveness of a dietary supplement. Eur Urol 2005;48(6):922–30, discussion 930–921.

[199] Ansari MS, Gupta NP. Lycopene: a novel drug therapy in hormone refractory metastatic prostate cancer. Urol Oncol 2004;22(5):415–20.

[200] Ansari MS, Gupta NP. A comparison of lycopene and orchidectomy vs orchidectomy alone in the management of advanced prostate cancer. BJU Int 2003;92(4):375–8, discussion 378.

[201] Jatoi A, Burch P, Hillman D, et al. A tomato-based, lycopene-containing intervention for androgen-independent prostate cancer: results of a Phase II study from the North Central Cancer Treatment Group. Urology 2007;69(2):289–94.

Hematol Oncol Clin N Am 22 (2008) 619–630

HEMATOLOGY/ONCOLOGY CLINICS
OF NORTH AMERICA

Review of Reliable Information Sources Related to Integrative Oncology

Kate Boddy, MA*, Edzard Ernst, MD, PhD, FRCP, FRCPEd

Complementary Medicine, Peninsula Medical School, Universities of Exeter and Plymouth, 25 Victoria Park Road, Exeter, EX2 4NT, UK

The sheer amount of information about complementary or alternative medicine (CAM) that is now available can be overwhelming. A simple Google search for the terms "complementary medicine or alternative medicine", conducted in January 2008, generated 1,300,000 hits, and this number grows on a daily basis. With such a vast amount of information available, how is one to know what is reliable and objective? Such a huge quantity of unregulated information inevitably leads to great variations in quality. Unfortunately, popularity is no guarantee; even the most commonly used integrative oncology Web sites offer information that is extremely variable in quality [1].

The information needs of both patient and health provider are very great, yet they are also very different. Both require accurate information to make informed decisions [2], but the type and style will vary greatly. Clinicians need to be certain the information they are accessing is reliable; they also need help finding this information. Tan and colleagues [3] interviewed oncology clinicians and found that the barriers they faced when accessing online cancer information were environmental, personal, and economic. Therefore, clinicians would be helped by a pre-evaluated list of reliable sources to overcome these barriers.

Clinicians need to know about good quality information sources, not only for themselves but also for their patients; healthcare professionals are the most frequently used source of information by oncology patients [4–6]. Yet according to Dooley [7], "there is little data regarding the sources of clinical information on CAM that oncology practitioner utilise." Dooley surveyed oncologists about their CAM information-seeking behaviors and found that the usefulness and reliability of the sources they accessed were inconsistent.

Clinicians should be able to guide patients to reliable sources [2]. Research shows that access to good-quality reliable information can ease the burden of worry suffered by patients [8]. Health care providers need to be familiar with the information sources their patients may be accessing [9] and vigilant

*Corresponding author. E-mail address: k.boddy@ex.ac.uk (K. Boddy).

0889-8588/08/$ – see front matter
doi:10.1016/j.hoc.2008.04.004

to the dangers of unreliable information. The Internet is the most frequently used mass media source by patients [2,4,10,11]. Patients generally tend to trust information they have retrieved from the Internet. Clinicians, however, are more wary of this source; in a survey conducted by Newnham [12], 91% of oncology health professionals believed that information found on the Internet had the potential to cause harm to their patients. Research has confirmed that health professionals are justified in their concerns. Analysis of Web sites providing information about CAM and cancer found that they "had the potential for harming patients" [1]. A more recent study analyzing content quality of pediatric neuro-oncology Web sites, found that 60% of sites were rated either poor or very poor [13].

AIM

The aim of this article is to provide an overview of reliable integrative oncology information from various resources. Clinical databases, research databases, online information systems, and print media were assessed for use by oncology health professionals and patients. The resources that are presented in this article provide high-quality information in keeping with an evidence-based approach to integrative medicine.

METHODS

Resource Selection

The resources listed have been selected for a critical review of information about evidence-based integrative oncology. Several criteria were employed to select reliable resources for this review:

1. An initial search was performed using the Intute database [14]. Intute is a free online service that provides access to pre-evaluated Web resources for education and research. All material were selected and evaluated by a network of subject specialists to create the database. Searches were conducted on the Web site using the keywords "integrative medicine, complementary medicine," and "alternative medicine". The first 20 results of each were saved for pre-evaluation.

2. A further search was performed using the Health on the Net (HON) Foundation online database [15]. The foundation promotes and guides the deployment of useful and reliable online medical and health information, and its appropriate and efficient use. Using its HON code system, over 5000 websites that provide quality online health information have been accredited. The keyword searches were repeated on this database, and the first 20 of each saved.

3. Sites then were evaluated using criteria described. The sites that achieved a high score on the evaluation scale were put forward for inclusion in this article. Because of space constraints, it was not possible to include all the high ranking resources in this article. The authors used their discretion to compile an article that provides a balance between databases, online information resources, and print media.

4. In addition to the previously mentioned selection procedures, the authors used their own expert knowledge to compile a list of integrative medicine organizations.

Resource Evaluation

The selected resources were evaluated using the DISCERN rating instrument [16]. DISCERN is a validated short questionnaire used to assess the quality of written information on treatment choices for health conditions. DISCERN has been designed to evaluate the reliability of information and assesses sources of evidence, currency, bias, and breadth, among other criteria. The scale provides a rating out of five, with one rated as "low quality: serious or extensive shortcomings," and five rated as "high quality: minimal shortcomings". Only material that was rated four or five on the scale was included in this article. The material in the Integrative Medicine Journals, Integrative Medicine Organizations, and Integrative Medicine Cancer Centers sections has not been subjected to a DISCERN evaluation, as the scale is not an appropriate measure for this type of resource.

This article is not an exhaustive list; space constraints mean that only a limited selection of resources could be included here. The selected resources usually contain links to additional information sources of high quality, and the databases provide plenty of linked material for further reading. The resources mentioned within this article are summarized in Table 1, with indications of who might find the resource most useful.

RESULTS

Review of Resources

Clinically oriented databases

The National Cancer Institute complementary and alternative medicine summaries. The National Cancer Institute's (NCI) Web site (www.cancer.gov/cancertopics/treatment/cam) contains a wealth of cancer-related information. A range of consumer-oriented information is available for the general public, patients, and health professionals, as well as comprehensive descriptions of the research programs and clinical trials the organization is undertaking. Information is available in English or Spanish. Summaries of various CAM treatments for cancer are provided on two levels, one for patients and one for health care professionals. The patient summaries avoid technical jargon, are easy to understand, and contain minimal references. They summarize the evidence and provide a bottom-line conclusion.

The health care professional summaries are very different. The professional summaries aim to provide comprehensive, peer-reviewed, evidence-based information about different CAM treatments. The summaries are intended to assist clinicians and other health professionals who work with cancer patients. They are complied and edited by an eminent board of United States CAM researchers and oncologists. Each summary begins with a quick glance that outlines the key facts and findings. Detailed general information about

Table 1
Summary of information resources

Name	Web site address	Who will find it most useful?
The National Cancer Institute complementary and alternative medicine summaries	www.cancer.gov/cancertopics/treatment/cam	Patients Researchers Clinicians
National Center for Complementary and Alternative Medicine	http://nccam.nih.gov	Patients
Natural standard, the authority on integrative medicine	http://www.naturalstandard.com/	Clinicians Researchers Patients
Allied and complementary medicine database	http://www.bl.uk/collections/health/amed.html	Researchers Clinicians
PubMed	http://pubmed.gov	Researchers Clinicians
The Cochrane library	http://www.mrw.interscience.wiley.com/cochrane/cochrane_search_fs.html	Researchers Clinicians
Office of Cancer Complementary and Alternative Medicine (OCCAM)	http://www.cancer.gov/cam/index.html	Clinicians Researchers
World Health Organization (WHO): traditional medicine	http://www.who.int/topics/traditional_medicine/en/	Clinicians Researchers
Society for Integrative Oncology	http://www.integrativeonc.org/	Clinicians Researchers
Consortium of academic health centers for integrative medicine	http://www.imconsortium.org/	Clinicians Researchers
International Society for Complementary Medicine Research	http://www.iscmr.org/index.html	Researchers Clinicians
The Research Council for Complementary Medicine	http://www.rccm.org.uk/	Researchers Clinicians
Memorial Sloan-Kettering Cancer Center	http://www.mskcc.org/mskcc/html/1979.cfm	Patients Clinicians
MD Anderson Cancer Center	http://www.mdanderson.org/departments/cimer/	Patients Clinicians
UK National Library for Complementary and Alternative Medicine Specialist	http://www.library.nhs.uk/cam/	Researchers Clinicians
Complementary and alternative medicine in the British Library's collections	http://www.bl.uk/collections/health/blcam.html	Researchers Clinicians

the treatment is followed by a history section. The summaries cover laboratory/animal and preclinical trials before detailing the human trials. Trials are described in detail. The last two sections of the summaries cover adverse effects and a conclusion based on the overall level of evidence. Each section is referenced very heavily, and where possible, the links are provided to the PubMed abstracts, enabling professionals to access the sources used to compile the summaries.

In addition, the summaries also contain tables outlining the key points of the trials: type of study, type of cancer, number of patients, and strongest benefit reported. Most usefully, the tables also provide a level of evidence score. The evidence score was designed by the NCI's Adult Treatment Editorial Board and allows trials to be ranked according to the statistical strength of the study design and scientific strength of the treatment outcomes.

The quality of the information on the site is excellent, but the breadth of coverage is quite limited; currently there are only 20 reviews. The Web site, however, provides details of many other sources of information; it links to other CAM information Web sites and provides links to a host of other cancer information sites.

It is very easy to assess the currency of the information, as dates of compilation and updates are provided. The introduction also states that the summaries are reviewed regularly and updated by the editorial board, increasing the professional's trust that he or she is accessing the most current information. While compiling this information, the authors noted that summary updates had been made extremely recently.

The NCI Web site rated very highly on the DISCERN rating scale, achieving a maximum 5 high score. This is an excellent source of information that will be of most use to researchers and professionals.

National Center for Complementary and Alternative Medicine. The National Center for Complementary and Alternative Medicine (NCCAM) is one of the 27 institutes and centers that make up the US National Institutes of Health. NCCAM describes itself as the United States federal government's lead agency for scientific research on CAM. NCCAM's Web site's (http://nccam.nih.gov) aim is to disseminate reliable and authoritative information about CAM to health professionals and the general public. In addition, the organization aims to train CAM researchers and to conduct rigorous scientific CAM research. It provides extensive information about CAM. The health information is split into five main sections" understanding CAM, being an informed consumer, additional features (including a live chat facility), links to other organizations, and most importantly condition and treatment topics. Some of this information is also available in Spanish. It is difficult to ascertain who exactly has written the summaries; the authors could not establish who made up the editorial team and thus could not gauge their qualifications.

The health topics begin with a selection of the most popular condition and treatment summaries. The user also has the choice of selecting from either a condition-specific or treatment-specific alphabetical list. Much of the cancer information links to the NCI complementary medicine patient summaries. The treatment summaries are consumer- orientated, with sections on finding a practitioner, what to expect during a treatment session, and costs. References are provided in these sections. Specific trials are not mentioned, however, and there is no allusion to evidence of efficacy. The summaries are current and updated with creation and modification dates available at the bottom of the pages.

The site generally can be considered reliable and trustworthy; it scored quite well on the DISCERN rating, although some areas were poor. Clinicians only should use it as an introductory information source; more detailed and useful information is available elsewhere. It is, however, very useful for patients, as it provides a considerable amount of consumer advice, and health professionals would be able to recommend it confidently.

Natural Standard, the authority on integrative medicine. Natural Standard calls itself the authority on integrative medicine and aims to be exactly this. Its goal is to provide impartial high-quality evidence-based CAM information. The Web site (http://www.naturalstandard.com) contains a vast wealth of information that is supplemented continually with new topic areas. The large multidisciplinary team of editors and writers ensures the objectivity and reliability of the material. The names and credentials of the editorial board are accessible and reassure the reader of the caliber and authority of the people associated with the project.

The review methodology is available on the Web site for transparency and reproducibility and contains details of the search strategy, selection criteria, and data analysis. Details of the review process also are described. Natural Standard uses it own validated grading scale for assessing the level of evidence to support efficacy of a given therapy for a specific indication. Evidence is graded from A to F according to the type of evidence available.

There is a huge amount of information on the Web site, but it is very easy to navigate because of the excellent layout and organization. The homepage allows access to the databases that are of primary interest to oncology health professionals: Foods, Herbs and Supplements, Health and Wellness, and Medical Conditions. Each database contains hundreds of subject headings. Clicking on a subject heading within the databases, such as mistletoe, gives one a choice of four levels of information. The professional monograph is a comprehensive evidence-based systematic review. It covers efficacy, adverse effects, interactions, pregnancy/lactation, pharmacology/toxicology, dosing/standardization, and products tested by third-party laboratories. In addition, it includes evidence tables, statistical analysis, and quality rating of available clinical trials. The professional monographs are referenced extensively with links to the abstracts on PubMed. The bottom-line monograph could be used by patients and health professionals and offer a concise evidence-based review. The flashcard is intended to be used as a quick reference guide or patient handout and could also be useful as a handout for practitioners. There is also a news section providing the latest updates on a particular topic.

In addition to the main databases on therapies and conditions, there are two further databases on Comparative Effectiveness and Brand Names. The Comparative Effectiveness database is a very useful feature. It allows the user to choose a condition subject heading such as cancer, cancer pain, or a particular cancer type and immediately see the therapies ranked according to their evidence grading. Clicking on prostate cancer, for example, allows the user to see that only one CAM therapy is graded A; four are graded B, and the rest are C and below.

The Web site contains a host of supplementary items that will be of use to health care professionals. Under the heading Interactive Tools, various helpful features can be found such as an interactions checker, medical calculator, and a practitioner listing database among others. The Web site is accessible by institutional subscription only. For those who may not be able to subscribe, the main material of the Web site is also available in alternative formats such as a desktop version and a handheld version for an annual fee. They also have published the main herbs and supplements databases as textbooks.

The Natural Standard Web site scored very highly on the DISCERN scale, but there were a couple of areas that would have given it a maximum score if they were improved. First, although the databases are referenced heavily, the Web site does not offer any links to external organizations, other than PubMed. It may be that it is their policy not to endorse other Web sites or materials, but it is helpful, indeed essential, for health care professionals to be able to access supplementary information that is considered reliable. Second, it is very important to be able to establish the currency of the reviews. Modification dates on the Web site show that it is maintained and updated daily, but the reviews themselves do not contain created or updated dates. It would be helpful to know when a particular review was updated last.

These are, however, minor quibbles. The Natural Standard integrative medicine database is a vast, reliable, and authoritative resource and would be an asset to any health care professional.

Research-orientated databases
AMED–allied and complementary medicine database. AMED (http://www.bl.uk/col lections/health/amed.html) is a unique bibliographic database produced by the Health Care Information Service of the British Library. It is a research database consisting of bibliographic records from a range of publications. It references nearly 600 specialist and general journals in three separate subject areas: complementary medicine, palliative care, and several professions allied to medicine. The subject coverage for complementary medicine was begun in 1985, and most titles are in English. Most references from 1995 and later contain abstracts. Access, by means of various formats, is by subscription only, and details of the numerous subscription options are found on the British Library Web site [17]. A user's experience of the front end of the AMED database will

depend on the interface to which his or her organization has subscribed. The ease of searching and the accuracy also are determined by the interface used [18]. AMED is a useful resource for any health professional who wishes to access the scientific literature. Keyword searches are performed easily and will return substantial results from CAM specialist journals that usually are not included on PubMed.

PubMed. PubMed (http://pubmed.gov) is a freely accessible online bibliographical research database of biomedical journal citations and abstracts created by the US National Library of Medicine (NLM). Approximately 5000 journals published in more than 80 countries are indexed. A special feature of the database is that the records are indexed with NLM's controlled vocabulary, the Medical Subject Headings (MeSH). Detailed searching instructions are provided under the headings Help and Tutorials. Bastyr University Library has produced a useful guide to conducting CAM literature searches using PubMed [19]. It explores in detail the MeSH headings for CAM, looks at CAM keyword searching, and also explores the PubMed Complementary Medicine Subset feature. CAM on PubMed was developed jointly by the NLM and NCCAM to assist in the easy retrieval of journal articles related to various CAM therapies, approaches, and systems. The CAM subset feature can be found in the Limits section. As with all limiting search functions, caution should be applied when using it. It is important to do some preliminary search work before applying the limiter; otherwise important citations may be missed. Bastyr's guide provides further help in this area. Another useful subset is the cancer subset. This strategy uses terms from the neoplasms and related branches of MeSH, cancer-related text words, and MEDLINE journal titles. It was created jointly by NLM and the NCI to facilitate searching for subjects in all areas of cancer, ranging from clinical care to basic research.

A useful feature for any health professional who wants to find very good-quality evidence quickly is the Clinical Queries function. This allows one to choose either the Clinical Study Category to find citations corresponding to a specific clinical study category such as a randomized clinical trial, or the Systematic Reviews function that returns citations for systematic reviews, meta-analyses, reviews of clinical trials, evidence-based medicine, and guidelines.

PubMed provides a LinkOut feature, allowing users to link directly from PubMed to a range of information and services. LinkOut resources include full-text publications, biological databases, consumer health information, and research tools.

The Cochrane Library: evidence for health care decision making. The Cochrane Collaboration is an international nonprofit organization that aims to provide up-to-date information about the effects of health care. Its aim is to ensure health care decision making around the world is informed by high-quality research evidence. The Cochrane Library (http://www.mrw.interscience.wiley.com/cochrane_search_fs.html) itself is a collection of databases that contain high-quality, independent evidence. The Cochrane reviews represent the highest level of evidence on which to base clinical treatment decisions and internationally Cochrane reviews are considered to be the gold-standard in evidence-based health care. The library also provides other sources of reliable information, such as other systematic review abstracts, technology assessments, economic evaluations, and individual clinical trials.

The review teams are organized according to condition and are made up of internationally renowned researchers. The objectivity of the Cochrane steering group can be assessed, as it publishes full details of any financial interests or potential conflicts of interest.

Information can be searched for using the online search facility. Searches can be limited to a specific evidence type such as a Cochrane review, clinical trial, or health technology assessment, among others. Keywords can be limited by abstract, author or other category.

The Cochrane Database contains hundreds of systematic reviews on CAM. A quick search using the term "acupuncture" and limited to Cochrane systematic reviews returned 169 reviews. The site is well-organized and easy to navigate, and it scored very highly on the DISCERN scale. This is an excellent resource for health professionals needing gold-standard evidence about integrative medicine.

Integrative medicine journals
There are many journals that will be useful to those interested in integrative oncology. Journals range in scope and coverage from general (eg, *Evidence-Based Complementary and Alternative Medicine*), specific (eg, *Integrative Cancer Therapies*), and review (*Focus on Alternative and Complementary Therapies*). A useful tool to gauge the depth and breadth of the journal coverage available is the online journals ranking site SCImago Journal & Country Rank [20]. It is a portal that includes the journals and country scientific indicators developed from the information contained in Elsevier's Scopus database. It does not cover all CAM journals, but it gives an indication of the types of CAM journals available and ranks them according to its own prestige calculation.

The British Library has created a Web page that collates various Internet, database, and print resources on CAM [21]. It lists some key CAM journals and provides a brief summary of their aims and links to the journal Web sites. Further lists of CAM journals can be found on the UK National Library for Health Web site. Details of the journals with links to their homepages are contained within the Complementary and Alternative Medicine Specialist Library subsection [22].

Integrative medicine organizations
Office of Cancer Complementary and Alternative Medicine. The Office of Cancer Complementary and Alternative Medicine (OCCAM) coordinates the activities of the NCI regarding CAM. Its mission is to improve the quality of care of cancer patients, as well as those at risk for cancer and those recovering from cancer treatment. It does this by contributing to the advancement of evidence-based CAM practice and the sciences that support it as well as the availability of high-quality information for the health care community, researchers, and the general public.

The Web site (http://www.cancer.gov/cam/index/html) has a helpful Frequently Asked Questions section about OCCAM and CAM in general. The site contains information about clinical trials, news and events, research, and health.

World Health Organization: traditional medicine. The World Health Organization (WHO) traditional medicine Web site (http://www.who.int/topics/traditional_ medicine/en) provides links to descriptions of activities, reports, news and events, and contacts and cooperating partners in the various WHO programs and offices working in the field. Links to related Web sites and topics also are featured. Fact sheets on traditional medicine and safety are provided in printer-friendly formats.

Society for integrative oncology. The society is a nonprofit, multidisciplinary organization of respected professionals dedicated to studying and facilitating cancer treatment and the recovery process through the use of integrated therapeutic options. The society's aim is to educate oncology professionals, patients, and caregivers about the scientific validity, clinical benefits, toxicities, and limitations of current integrative therapies.

The Web site (http://www.integrativeonc.org) contains information about the society's goals and provides information about its officers. Details about forthcoming conferences and events and the society's journals also are supplied.

Consortium of academic health centers for integrative medicine. The consortium's aim is to help transform medicine and health care through rigorous scientific studies, new models of clinical care, and innovative educational programs that integrate biomedicine, the complexity of human beings, the intrinsic nature of healing, and the rich diversity of therapeutic systems. The association is comprised of 39 academic medical centers in the United States and Canada. The consortium has a strong subgroup on integrative oncology.

The Web site (http://www.imconsortium.org) contains information about the consortium members, details of conferences and events, integrative medicine resources, job opportunities, joining information, and a useful frequently asked questions section.

International Society for Complementary Medicine Research. The International Society for Complementary Medicine Research (http://www.iscmr.org/index.html) is an international scientific organization of researchers, practitioners, and policy makers that encourages complementary and integrative medicine research and provides a platform for knowledge and information exchange to enhance international communication and collaboration. They aim to make communication and collaboration among researchers and practitioners with an interest in research on a worldwide basis possible. The society organizes an annual complementary medicine research conference, produces a newsletter, and offers discounts on some CAM journals to its members.

The Research Council for Complementary Medicine. The aims of the UK Research Council for Complementary Medicine (RCCM) are to develop and extend

Table 2
Key features of the integrative medicine cancer centers

Cancer center	Web site address	Key features
Memorial Sloan-Kettering Cancer Center	http://www.mskcc.org/mskcc/html/1979.cfm	Evidence-based herbs, botanicals, supplements database Information about clinical trials Resource links
MD Anderson Cancer Center	http://www.mdanderson.org/departments/cimer/	Extensive evidence-based therapy reviews Information about clinical trials Extensive further information resource Mandarin Chinese or Spanish options

the evidence base for complementary medicine to provide practitioners and patients with information about the effectiveness of specific therapies and the treatment of particular conditions. There is extensive information available on the Web site (http://www.rccm.org.uk/), including, CAM book reviews, news and events, and details of the RCCM's current projects. The Useful Links section contains extensive information about CAM databases, CAM journals, and Cochrane reviews. The RCCM has developed The Complementary and Alternative Medicine Evidence Online (CAMEOL) database, which reviews research evidence of the effectiveness of several specific therapies within condition areas that are on the UK National Health Service Priority; these include cancer. Access to this database is by means of the RCCM homepage.

Integrative medicine cancer centers
Some of the large cancer centers offer integrative medicine services, and their Web sites can be very informative. Health professionals and patients may find useful information about treatment options to help in shared decision making. Two of the most informative Web sites are mentioned in Table 2.

SUMMARY

Clinicians and patients require access to information about integrative oncology that is objective and trustworthy. Patients and care providers rely on health care professionals to provide most of this information. Therefore, health care professionals need to be familiar with a range of resources. This article summarized some of the excellent resources available for integrative oncology in an attempt to address this information need.

References
[1] Schmidt K, Ernst E. Assessing Web sites on complementary and alternative medicine for cancer. Ann Oncol 2004;15(5):733–42.

[2] Newnham GM, Burns WI, Snyder RD, et al. Information from the Internet: attitudes of Australian oncology patients. Intern Med J 2006;36(11):718–23.

[3] Tan EL, Stark H, Lowinger JS, et al. Information sources used by New South Wales cancer clinicians: a qualitative study. Intern Med J 2006;36(11):711–7.

[4] Cowan C, Hoskins R. Information preferences of women receiving chemotherapy for breast cancer. Eur J Cancer Care (Engl) 2007;16(6):543–50.

[5] Chen X, Siu LL. Impact of the media and the internet on oncology: survey of cancer patients and oncologists in Canada. J Clin Oncol 2001;19(23):4291–7.

[6] Carlsson M. Cancer patients seeking information from sources outside the health care system. Support Care Cancer 2000;8(6):453–7.

[7] Dooley MJ, Lee DY, Marriott JL. Practitioners' sources of clinical information on complementary and alternative medicine in oncology. Support Care Cancer 2004;12(2):114–9.

[8] Booth K, Beaver K, Kitchener H, et al. Women's experiences of information, psychological distress, and worry after treatment for gynaecological cancer. Patient Educ Couns 2005;56(2):225–32.

[9] Vapiwala N, Mick R, Hampshire MK, et al. Patient initiation of complementary and alternative medical therapies (CAM) following cancer diagnosis. Cancer J 2006;12(6):467–74.

[10] Peterson MW, Fretz PC. Patient use of the Internet for information in a lung cancer clinic. Chest 2003;123(2):452–7.

[11] Shen J, Andersen R, Albert PS, et al. Use of complementary/alternative therapies by women with advanced-stage breast cancer. BMC Complement Altern Med 2002;2:8.

[12] Newnham GM, Burns WI, Snyder RD, et al. Attitudes of oncology health professionals to information from the Internet and other media. Med J Aust 2005;183(4):197–200.

[13] Hargrave DR, Hargrave UA, Bouffet E. Quality of health information on the internet in pediatric neuro-oncology. Neuro Oncol 2006;8(2):175–82.

[14] Intute. About intute. Available at: http://www.intute.ac.uk/about.html. Accessed January 30, 2008.

[15] Health on the Net Foundation. HON databases. Available at: http://www.hon.ch/. Accessed January 30, 2008.

[16] Discern. Discern online. Available at: http://www.discern.org.uk/. Accessed January 29, 2008.

[17] British Library. Available at: http://www.bl.uk/collections/health/amed.html. Accessed January 30, 2008.

[18] Younger P, Boddy K. A comparison of AMED search results via EBSCOhost, ovid, and dialog interfaces. Health Info Libr (under review).

[19] Bastyr University. Complementary and alternative medicine (CAM) research using medline. Available at: http://www.bastyr.edu/library/resources/researchguide/cammedline.asp. Accessed January 29, 2008.

[20] SCImago. SJR-SCImago journal and country rank. Available at: http://www.scimagojr.com. Accessed January 29, 2008.

[21] British Library. Complementary and alternative medicine in the British Library's collections. Available at: http://www.bl.uk/collections/health/blcam.html. Accessed January 29, 2008.

[22] National Library for Health. Complementary and alternative medicine specialist library. Available at: http://www.library.nhs.uk/cam/Page.aspx?pagename=JOURNALS. Accessed January 29, 2008.

Hematol Oncol Clin N Am 22 (2008) 631–648

HEMATOLOGY/ONCOLOGY CLINICS
OF NORTH AMERICA

The Value of Acupuncture in Cancer Care

Weidong Lu, MB, MPH, Lic Ac[a,b],
Elizabeth Dean-Clower, MD, MPH[a,b],
Anne Doherty-Gilman, MPH[b], David S. Rosenthal, MD[a,b,c],*

[a]Harvard Medical School, Boston, MA, USA
[b]Leonard P. Zakim Center for Integrative Therapies, Dana-Farber Cancer Institute, 44 Binney Street, Boston, MA 02115, USA
[c]Harvard University, Boston, MA, USA

In the United States, acupuncture is used to treat various symptoms and conditions associated with cancer and the adverse effects of cancer treatments. Several cancer centers in the United States, including Dana-Farber Cancer Institute (DFCI) in Boston, Memorial Sloan-Kettering Cancer Center in New York, and M.D. Anderson Cancer Center in Houston, are integrating acupuncture into cancer care. This trend parallels a broader trend of increasing use of complementary and alternative medicine (CAM) among cancer patients, estimated in some surveys to range between 48% and 83% [1–4]. Specific use of acupuncture by cancer patients is estimated to range between 1.7% and 31% [5–7]. Despite interest by conventional care providers and the public in the integration of acupuncture into cancer care, the full extent to which acupuncture can be applied to oncology care is limited by research evidence regarding its efficacy and safety in treating and preventing cancer-related symptoms.

There are a few conditions for which sound research has demonstrated acupuncture to be an effective and safe adjunct therapy for cancer care. Randomized clinical trials (RCT) have demonstrated that acupuncture is effective for chemotherapy-induced nausea and vomiting [8–10]. Research studies also suggest acupuncture may be helpful in managing cancer-related pain [11], chemotherapy-related neutropenia [12], cancer fatigue [13], and radiation-induced xerostomia [14–16].

Acupuncture, an ancient medical treatment originating in China, is gaining momentum and acceptance as a valid intervention in medical practice. In the past decade, acupuncture and other integrative medicine programs have

This work was supported by Grant No. 1K01AT004415-01 from the National Institutes of Health.

*Corresponding author. Dana-Farber Cancer Institute, 44 Binney Street, Boston, MA 02115. E-mail address: drose@uhs.harvard.edu (D.S. Rosenthal).

been established in many major medical centers in the United States. For example, in November 2000, the Leonard P. Zakim Center for Integrative Therapies (Zakim Center) was established at DFCI, a teaching hospital of Harvard Medical School, to provide complementary therapies to patients of DFCI. The Zakim Center is named in memory of Lenny Zakim, a cancer patient and advocate for an integrative approach to cancer treatment. The mission of the center is to educate and empower patients and staff by integrating the practice of complementary therapies into traditional cancer treatments. The National Institutes of Health (NIH) has defined acupuncture as

> "a family of procedures involving stimulation of anatomic locations on the skin by a variety of techniques. The most studied mechanism of stimulation of acupuncture points uses penetration of the skin by thin, solid, metallic needles, which are manipulated manually or by electrical stimulation" [17].

Currently, traditional Chinese medicine (TCM) serves as the most prevalent theoretic framework guiding the clinical practice of acupuncture in the United States, in which clinical decisions are based mainly upon the unique clinical patterns that conform to TCM theory. To integrate acupuncture into conventional medical practice successfully, it is critical to develop scientific, evidence-based knowledge of acupuncture through basic and clinical research.

There has been an increase in acupuncture research in the field of oncology in the past 20 years, especially since the 1997 NIH consensus conference on acupuncture [17]. This trend is reflected in the number of acupuncture research articles published on PubMed [18]. From 1987 to 2007, PubMed published 8,276 articles that were related to acupuncture, and 320 were specific to acupuncture in oncology. PubMed publications in 2007 grew 96% since 1987. Similarly, acupuncture articles increased 157% from the 323 published in 1987 to 876 released as of the first quarter of 2007, and acupuncture in oncology articles grew $3\frac{1}{2}$ times, from 12 to 42. Over this 20-year period, the United States and China published 68 (26%) and 66 (25%) of 255 articles related to acupuncture and oncology, respectively. For the United States, 53 (78%) of the 68 articles were released in the past 7 years. The United Kingdom was next most prolific, having released 21 (8%) of the 255 articles. Although absolute numbers remain small, the number of RCTs also has risen significantly in past years, with 10 studies primarily focused on nausea and vomiting (30%) and four (12%) on cancer-related pain. Seven (21%) articles from China focused on acupuncture's anesthetic role in cancer-related surgery. Although there were 12 (36%) of the 33 conducted trials on various cancers, seven (21%) were specific to breast cancer. Overall 63% of the studies reported positive results.

The rise in interest in acupuncture trials could be attributed not only to the NIH's consensus conference, but also to the increase in federal funding for CAM research since 1999.

MECHANISM OF ACTION

The mechanism of action of acupuncture has been of great interest to many researchers. Numerous mechanistic studies of acupuncture in animal models and people suggest that the effect of acupuncture is based primarily on stimulation to and the responses of the neuroendocrine system involving the central and peripheral nervous systems.

Data from animal research suggests that therapeutic acupuncture is mediated partially through opioidergic and/or monoaminergic neurotransmission involving the brainstem, thalamus, hypothalamic, and pituitary function [19–24]. Human neuroimaging data from functional MRI (fMRI), positron emission tomography (PET), and electroencephalography (EEG) have demonstrated that acupuncture stimulation moderates a wide network of brain regions, including the primary somatosensory, secondary somatosensory, and anterior cingulated, prefrontal, and insular cortices, amygdala, hippocampus, hypothalamus, and other areas [25–32]. The brain response may differ depending on *de qi*. *De qi* is a sensation experienced during acupuncture by the acupuncturist during the needle manipulation and by the patient who feels soreness, fullness, heaviness, local distension, or other sensations [28] at local needling sites [33]. A pilot study using fMRI suggests a relationship between stimulation of an acupuncture point, LI-2, located at the base of the index finger, and the activation of the brain function area that is responsible for salivary production, suggesting neural transmission [34].

In several animal models, acupuncture and other stimulation methods of acupuncture points, such as thread implantation and point injection, suggest that acupuncture could down-regulate the expression of transforming growth factor (TGF). Particularly, two independent studies on rat models of liver fibrosis and chronic renal failure found an inhibition of TGF-β1 expression in the tissues after acupuncture points were stimulated by either a thread implantation or injection with Chinese herbs [35,36].

It has been suggested that acupuncture stimulates production of granulocyte colony-stimulating factor (G-CSF) and granulocyte-macrophage colony-stimulating factor (GM-CSF) in animal models treated with myelosuppressive chemotherapy [37,38]. In one controlled nonrandomized human clinical trial, seven patients undergoing chemotherapy were treated with a course of nine daily acupuncture treatments. The serum G-CSF levels were measured before and after acupuncture treatment. There was a significant increase in G-CSF levels after acupuncture ($P < .001$), along with an increase in white blood cell (WBC) count level ($P < .01$) in this group of patients [38].

PLACE OF ACUPUNCTURE IN CLINICAL CANCER CARE

Recent advances in acupuncture clinical research suggest that acupuncture may provide clinical benefit for cancer patients with treatment-related adverse effects such as nausea and vomiting, postoperative pain, cancer-related pain, chemotherapy-induced leukopenia, postchemotherapy fatigue, xerostomia, and possibly insomnia, anxiety, and quality of life (QOL) (Table 1).

Table 1
Clinical trials and systematic review of acupuncture use in clinical cancer care (2001–2007)

Clinical conditions	Author and study design	Major outcome	Reported adverse events	Study population features
Chemotherapy-induced nausea and vomiting	Roscoe et al [9] randomized controlled multicenter trial (n = 739)	Patients in the acupressure group experienced less nausea on the day of treatment compared with controls ($P < .05$)	No adverse events were discussed	85% breast cancer, 10% hematologic neoplasms; patients undergoing chemotherapy
Postoperative nausea and vomiting	Gan et al [43] randomized clinical trial (RCT) (n = 77) (electro-acupoint stimulation, ondansetron versus placebo)	The complete response rate was 77% versus 64% and 42% ($P = .01$); electro-acupoint stimulation is more effective in controlling nausea	No difference in adverse events rate among groups	Patients undergoing major breast surgery
Cancer pain	Alimi et al [11] randomized, blinded, controlled trial (n = 90)	Pain intensity deceased by 36% at 2 months from baseline in the study group ($P < .0001$)	No infection was reported; no other adverse events were reported	Patients who have chronic peripheral or central neuropathic pain arising after cancer treatment
Postoperative pain	Mehling et al [62] RCT (n = 138) (Massage, acupuncture, usual care versus usual care alone)	Patients in the massage and acupuncture group who had usual care experienced a decrease of 1.4 points on a pain scale ($P = .038$)	No adverse events were discussed	Patients undergoing cancer-related surgery including breast, bladder, prostate, and ovarian cancers
Post-thoracotomy wound pain	Wong et al [61] RCT (n = 27) (electro-acupuncture versus sham acupuncture)	A trend for lower visual analog scale pain score in the electro-acupuncture group was observed. Postoperative morphine use was significantly lower in electro-acupuncture group ($P < .05$)	No adverse reactions related to acupuncture were observed	Patients who have operable nonsmall cell lung carcinoma

Symptom	Study	Results	Adverse effects	Population
Hot flashes	Deng et al [73] RCT (n = 72) (true acupuncture versus sham acupuncture)	True acupuncture was associated with 0.8 fewer hot flashes per day than sham (P = .3)	Very minor slight bleeding and bruising at the needle site were reported	Breast cancer patients
Vasomotor symptoms (hot flashes) and psychological well-being	Nedstrand et al [74] RCT (electro-acupuncture versus applied relaxation) (n = 38)	Longitudinally, patients in the electro-acupuncture group experienced a decrease of hot flashes >50% at 12 weeks and at 6 months follow-up	No adverse events were discussed	Patients treated for breast cancer
Chemotherapy-induced leukopenia	Lu et al [12] systematic review on RCTs (n = 682)	WBC counts in study group were significantly higher than that in control group (P < .05)	No adverse effects were discussed	Patients who have nonsmall cell lung cancer or nasopharynx cancer undergoing chemotherapy
Postchemotherapy fatigue	Vickers et al [13] uncontrolled prospective study (n = 37)	The mean improvement from baseline fatigue score was 31.3% (95% CI: 20.6%–41.5%)	No adverse events were reported	Cancer patients who had completed cytotoxic chemotherapy at least 3 weeks previously but complained of persisting fatigue
Radiation-induced xerostomia	Johnstone et al [15] uncontrolled prospective study (n = 50)	Response rate as improvement of 10% or better from baseline; xerostomia inventory (XI) was 70%; 48% of patients received benefit of 10 points or more on the XI	No adverse effects were reported	Patients who have pilocarpine-resistant xerostomia after radiotherapy for head and neck cancer

Chemotherapy-Induced Nausea and Vomiting

After the NIH Consensus Conference in 1997, several well-designed clinical trials generated promising results. A randomized controlled trial further confirmed acupuncture's antiemetic effect on patients receiving chemotherapy, with a significant reduction of mean emesis episodes (5 versus 15; $P < .001$) compared with pharmacotherapy alone [10]. The results of the study confirmed the NIH consensus statement about acupuncture:

> "There is clear evidence that needle acupuncture is efficacious for adult postoperative and chemotherapy nausea and vomiting and probably for the nausea of pregnancy" [17].

Methods other than acupuncture needles used to stimulate acupuncture points also have been reported to have a positive effect. These stimulating methods include manual acupressure, a non-needling procedure with manual pressure on acupuncture points, acupressure wrist bands with or without electrical stimulation, and ear acupuncture [9,39–41]. For example, acupressure wrist bands have shown positive results in controlling chemotherapy-induced nausea and vomiting in a large multicenter study [9]. Another study, however, indicated that using invasive needle acupuncture at P6, an antiemesis point, showed no additional effect for the prevention of acute nausea and vomiting in high-dose chemotherapy, compared with nonskin-penetrating placebo acupuncture [42]. In addition to chemotherapy-induced nausea and vomiting, acupuncture has been shown to be effective for preventing postoperative nausea and vomiting [43].

The authoritative Cochrane systematic review on this subject states that

> "data on postoperative nausea and vomiting suggest a biologic effect of acupuncture point stimulation. Electro-acupuncture has demonstrated benefit for chemotherapy-induced acute vomiting, but studies combining electro-acupuncture with state-of-the-art antiemetics and in patients with refractory symptoms are needed to determine clinical relevance. Self-administered acupressure appears to have a protective effect for acute nausea and readily can be taught to patients though studies did not involve placebo control. Noninvasive electrostimulation appears unlikely to have a clinically relevant impact when patients are given state-of-the-art pharmacologic antiemetic therapy" [44].

Cancer Pain

Pain is a long-standing and unresolved clinical issue among patients who have cancer. Even after over 20 years since the World Health Organization (WHO) published its recommendation of an analgesic ladder for pain control [45], 55% of patients who have cancer still suffer from various forms of pain that significantly impact their QOL [46]. One of the reported barriers is the resistance to start opioid therapy either by the patient or the physician [47]. Alternatively, inappropriate use of opioids is associated with significant adverse effects among patients who have cancer [48].

Acupuncture analgesia has been studied actively in the laboratory and clinic for several decades. Several systematic reviews support the use of acupuncture for a range of noncancer specific pain conditions in clinical practice. These pain conditions include osteoarthritis [49], chronic knee pain [50,51], shoulder pain [52], neck pain [53], and acute dental pain [54]. Although the numbers of acupuncture clinical trials for cancer-specific pain are still small, results of these noncancer-related clinical trials may support benefit for patients who have cancer. First, cancer pain may be brought on by a combination of biological, psychological, and social components [55]. Acupuncture-induced analgesic effects can influence the psychological aspect of pain strongly [56]. Second, because most patients who have cancer are in the older population, a stage when significant numbers are reported to have chronic pain, pain reported from patients who have cancer may not necessarily be directly cancer-related and may respond to acupuncture. Third, several RCTs specifically studied acupuncture pain control during surgical procedures and found that acupuncture reduced analgesic requirement of drugs such as morphine, piritramide, and alfentanil [57–60]. Therefore, it is reasonable to believe that acupuncture could serve as a nonpharmaceutical mediator to assist the WHO analgesic ladder for cancer pain.

In the field of cancer-specific pain management, a randomized placebo-controlled trial demonstrated that auricular acupuncture is effective for cancer patients with various forms of neuropathic pain [11]. Several other randomized controlled clinical trials have suggested that acupuncture can be used for the following conditions to manage pain among cancer patients:

Chronic constant neuropathic pain in postcancer therapies [11]
Post-thoracotomy pain in patients who have operable nonsmall cell lung carcinoma [61]
Other postoperative pain in patients who have breast cancer, bladder cancer, prostate cancer, and ovarian cancer [62]

In these clinical settings, acupuncture often is used as a complementary method along with usual care to provide additional pain reduction, and to lessen the need for pharmaceutical analgesic medicine.

SYMPTOM RELIEF
Depression and Anxiety
A recently published RCT reports that massage combined with acupuncture in postoperative cancer patients can improve the depressive mood of these patients when used in conjunction with usual care ($P = .003$). A short-lived improvement in tension and anxiety also was found in this study ($P = .048$) [62].

Although conducted in noncancer patients, several RCTs have found that acupuncture may reduce patient anxiety significantly during acute physical trauma (eg, radial fractures, hip fracture), hospital transportation, during or before lithotripsy and dental procedures, and cataract surgery [63–68]. In addition to acupuncture needle stimulation on traditional body acupuncture points, ear acupuncture, ear acupressure, and acupressure on other body parts also seem to be effective in providing mild-to-moderate sedative effects in anxious patients [69–71].

Hot Flashes

Using acupuncture for hot flashes in patients who have breast cancer is another active area of clinical study. Although empiric reports suggest that acupuncture is beneficial to reduce the number of hot flashes in patients who have breast cancer [72], a recently published well-controlled clinical trial failed to demonstrate the benefit of active acupuncture as compared with sham acupuncture in reducing hot flashes [73]. Interestingly, hot flash frequency in breast cancer patients in this study was reduced following both true and sham acupuncture. The authors suggest that a longer and more intense acupuncture intervention could produce a larger reduction in all of these symptoms [73]. Another less rigorous RCT from Sweden reported a more than 50% reduction of hot flashes and other associated symptoms in breast cancer patients after receiving a 12-week electro-acupuncture intervention [74]. There was a suggestion in this study that the symptom reduction effect was durable, lasting up to 6 months.

Leukopenia

Although there is an absence of medical literature in the English language on the use acupuncture for leukopenia, several RCTs conducted in China have suggested that acupuncture could be effective in reducing marrow suppression-related leukopenia in patients undergoing chemotherapy [75–77]. An exploratory meta-analysis of clinical trials conducted in China suggests that acupuncture use is associated with an increase in leukocytes in patients during chemotherapy or chemo-radiotherapy, with a weighted mean difference of 1221 white blood cells (WBC)/μL on average (95% CI 636 to 1807; $P < .0001$) [12]. A randomized sham-controlled clinical trial exploring chemotherapy-induced neutropenia in ovarian cancer patients has been completed at DFCI, and preliminary data suggest improved neutrophil counts at the nadir and rebound points after chemotherapy [78,79].

Fatigue

Several prospective pilot trials have shown acupuncture may benefit patients who have chemotherapy-related fatigue [13,80]. In patients with persistent fatigue who previously had completed cytotoxic therapy and were not anemic, acupuncture resulted in a 31.3% improvement in the baseline fatigue score [13].

Neuropathy

Chemotherapy-induced neuropathy eg, from platinum- and taxol-related compounds, is a common problem. A small pilot study of five patients suggested a partial response to acupuncture that could not be explained by any other known neurophysiologic mechanism [81]. A positive impact from acupuncture on neuropathy in DFCI clinic patients also has been observed.

Insomnia

Insomnia is one of the most significant symptoms of patients who have cancer, along with anxiety. Acupuncture has been researched among patients with insomnia with mixed results. A small, noncancer study found acupuncture may reduce insomnia and anxiety significantly, with clear objective improvements in nocturnal melatonin secretion and in polysomnographic measures [66]. A meta-analysis showed that the improvement rate of insomnia produced by ear acupuncture was significantly higher than those from diazepam ($P < .05$) [82]. The rate of success was particularly higher when ear acupuncture was used for enhancement of sleeping hours, up to 6 hours in treatment subjects ($P < .05$). The authors of this study concluded that ear acupuncture appears to be effective for treating insomnia.

In a Cochrane systematic review of acupuncture for insomnia, however, the authors found that acupuncture or its variants were not more significantly effective than a control (relative risk (RR) = 1.66, 95% CI = 0.68 to −4.03) [83]. According to the authors, "The current evidence is not sufficiently extensive or rigorous enough to support the use of any form of acupuncture for treating insomnia." Larger high-quality clinical trials employing appropriate randomization, concealment, and blinding with longer follow-up are warranted to further investigate the efficacy and safety of acupuncture for treating insomnia.

Radiation-Induced Xerostomia

Xerostomia, or dry mouth, is considered a significant factor underlying dysphagia. Several pilot clinical studies suggest that acupuncture may improve xerostomia caused by radiation therapy in patients who have head and neck cancers. Blom first reported a small RCT with placebo acupuncture control in which acupuncture treatment induced a persistent salivary flow rate among a group of patients who had severe xerostomia. A long-term follow up (up to 32 months) further confirmed his findings [14,84,85]. Johnstone and colleagues [15,86] used acupuncture for patients who had pilocarpine-resistant xerostomia after radiotherapy for head and neck cancer. They found a 70% response rate (ie, an increase of 10% or more from the baseline Xerostomia Inventory). Wong and colleagues [16] reported a phase 1–2 study using transcutaneous electrical stimulation. Forty-six patients were randomized among three groups with different acupuncture points. After 6 weeks of treatment, for 37 patients who completed the treatment course, the salivation increase was statistically significant at both 3- and 6-month follow-ups. Studies using fMRI found a relationship between stimulating acupuncture point, LI-2, located at the base of index finger, and the activation of the brain function area responsible for salivary production [34].

Dyspnea

Although clinical evidence for acupuncture treating dyspnea in patients who have cancer is yet to come, some preliminary RCTs suggest acupuncture and acupressure may improve respiratory function and QOL among patients who have chronic obstructive asthma, bronchiectasis, and chronic obstructive pulmonary disease [87–89]. Therefore, acupuncture/acupressure for dyspnea in patients who have cancer is a promising area for future studies.

Acupuncture in Palliative Care

A pilot study demonstrated feasibility of administering acupuncture as adjuvant palliative therapy to patients who have advanced cancer [90]. Forty ambulatory patients with advanced ovarian or breast cancer who were receiving conventional palliative care were recruited to receive acupuncture treatment for 8 weeks (12 sessions total). Twenty-six patients (65%) completed all 8 weeks of treatment, thereby achieving the study's main feasibility goal. Over time, a significant decrease in symptom severity was seen for fatigue, pain, and insomnia. QOL measures of pain severity and interference, physical and psychological distress, life satisfaction, and mood states showed higher positive scores during acupuncture treatment than before treatment and were sustained at 12 weeks relative to baseline. This pilot study warrants study in a larger population using proper controls.

CLINICAL PRACTICE

An important criterion to evaluate a therapy in clinical practice is the safety record of that therapy. Several studies on the safety of acupuncture have confirmed that acupuncture is a safe procedure in the hands of competent practitioners. One large study found only 43 minor adverse events associated with 34,407 treatments, with no serious adverse events reported [91]. Based upon the criteria proposed by Weiger and colleagues [92], in which the clinical effectiveness and the risk ratios of CAM therapies are weighed simultaneously, acupuncture for chemotherapy-related nausea and vomiting and for pain have been categorized as "safe and effective" and can be "recommended" as an adjunct to conventional therapy. The assurance of acupuncture safety is emphasized further by the US Food and Drug Administration regulation of acupuncture needles as a medical device [93], the training and licensing of clinical acupuncturists, and continuing education courses and licensing now available to physicians. Medicare has recognized acupuncture by assigning it current procedural terminology (CPT) codes, thereby promoting insurance and health expense account reimbursement.

Despite the wide use of CAM therapies among patients who have cancer and despite its safety and efficacy, acupuncture use in this population remains low. The prevalence of CAM use varied in range from 48% to 83% among patients who had cancer in several studies depending on the definition of CAM [1,2,4]. One recent study found that among insured cancer patients in Washington state, the acupuncture usage was only 1.7% in 2000 [6]. A survey among 1065 Chinese women who had breast cancer found that although 98% of patients had used at least one form of CAM therapy, the use rate of acupuncture was only 4.9% [5]. Similar findings were reported by Ganz (2.2%) and Burstein (4.0%) [94,95]. The highest use rate of acupuncture in patients who had cancer was reported by Morris and colleagues [7] as 31% of 617 responses. The use of acupuncture is associated with the economic status of patients, because it requires patients to consult a CAM practitioner whose services generally are not covered by health insurance companies. Although some major cancer centers now provide acupuncture services to cancer patients, the scale of such services remains small. The paucity of referrals from clinicians and the need to self-pay for the acupuncture are considered two main barriers for using acupuncture.

RESEARCH ISSUES

Clinical research of acupuncture in cancer care has been supported by federal and private funding sources. A steady increase in reports from high-quality clinical trials is expected in the next few years. This will help improve clinical decision-making about acupuncture, because current available results from many studies suffer from poor study design. The shortcomings of these clinical trials exist mainly in three areas: (1) the design of the clinical trial, (2) the quality control employed in conducting the trial, and (3) the complete, detailed reporting of the clinical trial. As a result, often study results are difficult to interpret. The design of clinical trials of acupuncture should comply with the general principles of clinical trials in medicine, such as adequate sample size, power calculations, randomization, and effective concealment of treatment assignment. Clinicians who have a background in pharmaceutical trials should be made fully aware of the uniqueness of acupuncture clinical studies.

In the past, most clinical trials of acupuncture were designed by clinicians who were not trained specifically in clinical trial design. Therefore, the quality of acupuncture trials was considerably poor. For example, many systematic reviews revealed that most trials reported randomization only, which is only one of three commonly recognized key domains in quality trials; blinding and handling of dropouts and withdrawals were not mentioned [12,83,96]. It is recognized that although quality scales are important tools to assess the integrity of clinical trials, they are poor surrogates of the true quality of a specific trial. Some studies suggested that the poor quality of a trial could lead to inflated results. Trials with inadequate concealment and ineffective blinding could lead to exaggerated odds ratios by 41% and 17%, respectively [97].

Although inappropriate design of clinical trials of acupuncture remains an issue of concern, many clinician scientists have begun to get involved in the design process of acupuncture trials. Lack of familiarity with acupuncture technique, however, and the assumption that an acupuncture clinical trial is exactly the same as a pharmaceutical trial potentially may lead to inaccurate results. Currently, the largest issue in clinical trials of acupuncture is the controversy of sham acupuncture as an effective control. Choosing the appropriate control for acupuncture clinical trials is a challenging task. Although several control methods are available, there remains a lack of consensus about which one is the most effective type of sham control [98–100]. As many researchers point out, an ideal sham control should mimic verum (true) acupuncture as much as possible, while at the same time not elicit any physiologic effect on the study subjects.

A placebo needle (Streiberger needle) has been used in many clinical trials of acupuncture, in which the needle mimics the sensation of needle insertion with its blunt tip and appears to penetrate the skin, but it actually retracts into a hollow shaft [101]. Many studies have reported that this needle produces a very high-quality and effective blinding effect on study patients [42,56]. Critics, however, point out that acupuncture essentially is based upon the sensation of needle insertion, *de qi*; while other types of acupuncture variations, such as acupressure and wrist bands, are not required to penetrate the skin, they still produce the *de qi* sensation to produce clinical results. Other sham acupuncture methods, such as superficial acupuncture needling, mock electro-acupuncture stimulation, needling at nonmeridians and nontraditional acupuncture points also have been used in many trials. These methods have their shortcomings and limitations also. Clinical trials have demonstrated that sham acupuncture has different effects on pain than a placebo pill [56]. A study of experimental pain processing also revealed that placebo needling may evoke different types of brain responses than those evoked by more conventional placebos, such as creams or pills [102].

The implementation of clinical trials of acupuncture is another important issue. Because acupuncture is essentially a procedure involving skilled hand manipulation that is highly dependent on the operator's experience and the technique used, minimizing the variations during acupuncture performance is a critical issue to ensure the success of the clinical trials. A careful and meticulous standardization of each procedure should be planned, and adequate training for such standardization should be provided before a trial starts.

Standards for Reporting Interventions in Controlled Trials of Acupuncture (STRICTA) [103], a Consolidated Standards of Reporting Trials-based recommendation on acupuncture trials, has been published. It focuses on complete reporting of interventions rather than a quality measure scale. Because of the nonpharmaceutical and procedure-like nature of acupuncture trials, a discipline-specific quality measure scale needs to be developed further.

SUMMARY

Clinical research on acupuncture in cancer care is a new and challenging field in oncology. The results of clinical research will continue to provide clinically relevant answers for patients and oncologists. The evidence currently available has suggested that acupuncture is a safe and effective therapy to manage cancer and treatment related symptoms, while giving patients the ability to actively participate in their own care plan.

Future research requires the involvement of clinical researchers, clinicians, and patients. Development of innovative research methods is also crucial. It is expected that as more evidence continues to emerge, oncology acupuncture eventually will be integrated into standard oncology practice. The successful integration of acupuncture at major academic medical and research facilities, such as DFCI and other major cancer centers, underscores the need for and value of acupuncture in cancer care.

References

[1] DiGianni LM, Garber JE, Winer EP. Complementary and alternative medicine use among women with breast cancer. J Clin Oncol 2002;20(Suppl 18):34S–38S.

[2] Ernst E, Cassileth BR. The prevalence of complementary/alternative medicine in cancer: a systematic review. Cancer 1998;83(4):777–82.

[3] Lee MM, Lin SS, Wrensch MR, et al. Alternative therapies used by women with breast cancer in four ethnic populations. J Natl Cancer Inst 2000;92(1):42–7.

[4] Richardson MA. Complementary and alternative therapy use in gynecologic oncology: implications for clinical practice. Gynecol Oncol 2002;84(3):360–2.

[5] Cui Y, Shu XO, Gao Y, et al. Use of complementary and alternative medicine by Chinese women with breast cancer. Breast Cancer Res Treat 2004;85(3):263–70.

[6] Lafferty WE, Bellas A, Corage Baden A, et al. The use of complementary and alternative medical providers by insured cancer patients in Washington state. Cancer 2004;100(7): 1522–30.

[7] Morris KT, Johnson N, Homer L, et al. A comparison of complementary therapy use between breast cancer patients and patients with other primary tumor sites. Am J Surg 2000;179(5):407–11.

[8] Dundee JW, Ghaly RG, Fitzpatrick KT, et al. Acupuncture prophylaxis of cancer chemotherapy-induced sickness. J R Soc Med 1989;82(5):268–71.

[9] Roscoe JA, Morrow GR, Hickok JT, et al. The efficacy of acupressure and acustimulation wrist bands for the relief of chemotherapy-induced nausea and vomiting. A University of Rochester Cancer Center Community Clinical Oncology Program multicenter study. J Pain Symptom Manage 2003;26(2):731–42.

[10] Shen J, Wenger N, Glaspy J, et al. Electro-acupuncture for control of myeloablative chemotherapy-induced emesis: a randomized controlled trial. JAMA 2000;284(21): 2755–61.

[11] Alimi D, Rubino C, Pichard-Leandri E, et al. Analgesic effect of auricular acupuncture for cancer pain: a randomized, blinded, controlled trial. J Clin Oncol 2003;21(22): 4120–6.

[12] Lu W, Hu D, Dean-Clower E, et al. Acupuncture for chemotherapy-induced leukopenia: exploratory meta-analysis of randomized controlled trials. J Soc Integr Oncol 2007;5(1): 1–10.

[13] Vickers AJ, Straus DJ, Fearon B, et al. Acupuncture for postchemotherapy fatigue: a phase II study. J Clin Oncol 2004;22(9):1731–5.

[14] Blom M, Dawidson I, Fernberg JO, et al. Acupuncture treatment of patients with radiation-induced xerostomia. Eur J Cancer B Oral Oncol 1996;32(3):182–90.

[15] Johnstone PA, Peng YP, May BC, et al. Acupuncture for pilocarpine-resistant xerostomia following radiotherapy for head and neck malignancies. Int J Radiat Oncol Biol Phys 2001;50(2):353–7.

[16] Wong RK, Jones GW, Sagar SM, et al. A Phase I–II study in the use of acupuncture-like transcutaneous nerve stimulation in the treatment of radiation-induced xerostomia in head-and-neck cancer patients treated with radical radiotherapy. Int J Radiat Oncol Biol Phys 2003;57(2):472–80.

[17] NIH Consensus Conference. Acupuncture. JAMA 1998;280(17):1518–24.

[18] Lu M, Doherty-Gilman A, Rosenthal DS, et al. Research articles published on PubMed in the field of acupuncture and acupuncture oncology from 1987 to 2007: trends in growth and international contribution. Presented at: Society for Integrative Oncology 4th International Conference. San Francisco, California, November 15–17, 2007.

[19] Han JS. Acupuncture: neuropeptide release produced by electrical stimulation of different frequencies. Trends Neurosci 2003;26(1):17–22.

[20] Han JS, Tang J, Ren MF, et al. Central neurotransmitters and acupuncture analgesia. Am J Chin Med 1980;8(4):331–48.

[21] Han JS, Xie GX, Zhou ZF, et al. Enkephalin and beta-endorphin as mediators of electro-acupuncture analgesia in rabbits: an antiserum microinjection study. Adv Biochem Psychopharmacol 1982;33:369–77.

[22] Han JS, Xie GX, Zhou ZF, et al. Acupuncture mechanisms in rabbits studied with microinjection of antibodies against beta-endorphin, enkephalin and substance P. Neuropharmacology 1984;23(1):1–5.

[23] Liang XB, Liu XY, Li FQ, et al. Long-term high-frequency electro-acupuncture stimulation prevents neuronal degeneration and up-regulates BDNF mRNA in the substantia nigra and ventral tegmental area following medial forebrain bundle axotomy. Brain Res Mol Brain Res 2002;108(1–2):51–9.

[24] Zhou ZF, Du MY, Wu WY, et al. Effect of intracerebral microinjection of naloxone on acupuncture and morphine analgesia in the rabbit. Sci Sin 1981;24(8):1166–78.

[25] Chen AC, Liu FJ, Wang L, et al. Mode and site of acupuncture modulation in the human brain: 3D (124-ch) EEG power spectrum mapping and source imaging. Neuroimage 2006;29(4):1080–91.

[26] Hsieh JC, Tu CH, Chen FP, et al. Activation of the hypothalamus characterizes the acupuncture stimulation at the analgesic point in human: a positron emission tomography study. Neurosci Lett 2001;307(2):105–8.

[27] Hui KK, Liu J, Makris N, et al. Acupuncture modulates the limbic system and subcortical gray structures of the human brain: evidence from fMRI studies in normal subjects. Hum Brain Mapp 2000;9(1):13–25.

[28] Hui KK, Liu J, Marina O, et al. The integrated response of the human cerebro-cerebellar and limbic systems to acupuncture stimulation at ST 36 as evidenced by fMRI. Neuroimage 2005;27(3):479–96.

[29] Kim MS, Nam TC. Electroencephalography (EEG) spectral edge frequency for assessing the sedative effect of acupuncture in dogs. J Vet Med Sci 2006;68(4):409–11.

[30] Litscher G. Effects of acupressure, manual acupuncture, and laser needle acupuncture on EEG bispectral index and spectral edge frequency in healthy volunteers. Eur J Anaesthesiol 2004;21(1):13–9.

[31] Napadow V, Makris N, Liu J, et al. Effects of electro-acupuncture versus manual acupuncture on the human brain as measured by fMRI. Hum Brain Mapp 2005;24(3):193–205.

[32] Wong VC, Sun JG, Yeung DW. Pilot study of positron emission tomography (PET) brain glucose metabolism to assess the efficacy of tongue and body acupuncture in cerebral palsy. J Child Neurol 2006;21(6):456–62.

[33] Langevin HM, Churchill DL, Fox JR, et al. Biomechanical response to acupuncture needling in humans. J Appl Physiol 2001;91(6):2471–8.

[34] Deng GE. Randomized controlled study of fMRI changes associated with acupuncture at a point used to treat xerostomia versus sham acupuncture or gustatory stimulation. Presented at the Society for Integrative Oncology 3rd International Conference. Boston, Massachusetts, November 9–11, 2006.

[35] Liu HR, Ma XF, Zhao TP, et al. Regulation of acupuncture & moxibustion on collagen and TGF-β mRNA in colon of Crohn's disease rats [in Chinese]. Journal of Anhui Tradiational Chinese Medicine College 2005;24(4):25–8.

[36] Zhou AL, Luo L, Zhou CH, et al. Effects of acupoint injection with oxymatrine on expression of type IV collagen and TGF-β1 mRNA on rat liver fibrosis [in Chinese]. Chinese Medical Journal of Communications 2005;19(5):421–4.

[37] Jiang D, Xu Y, Qi Z, et al. Effect of electro-acupuncture on peripheral leukocyte count, CFU-GM frequency and plasma cGMP level in rats. Bulletin of Hunan Medical University 1989;14(4):335–7.

[38] Zhao X, Wang H, Cao D, et al. Influence of acupuncture and moxibustion on serum CSF activity of patients with leukopenia caused by chemotherapy. Zhen Ci Yan Jiu 1999; 24(1):17–9.

[39] Dibble SL, Luce J, Cooper BA, et al. Acupressure for chemotherapy-induced nausea and vomiting: a randomized clinical trial. Oncol Nurs Forum 2007;34(4):813–20.

[40] Josefson A, Kreuter M. Acupuncture to reduce nausea during chemotherapy treatment of rheumatic diseases. Rheumatology (Oxford) 2003;42(10):1149–54.

[41] Molassiotis A, Helin AM, Dabbour R, et al. The effects of P6 acupressure in the prophylaxis of chemotherapy-related nausea and vomiting in breast cancer patients. Complement Ther Med 2007;15(1):3–12.

[42] Streitberger K, Friedrich-Rust M, Bardenheuer H, et al. Effect of acupuncture compared with placebo acupuncture at P6 as additional antiemetic prophylaxis in high-dose chemotherapy and autologous peripheral blood stem cell transplantation: a randomized controlled single-blind trial. Clin Cancer Res 2003;9(7):2538–44.

[43] Gan TJ, Jiao KR, Zenn M, et al. A randomized controlled comparison of electro-acupoint stimulation or ondansetron versus placebo for the prevention of postoperative nausea and vomiting. Anesth Analg 2004;99(4):1070–5, table of contents.

[44] Ezzo J, Vickers A, Richardson MA, et al. Acupuncture point stimulation for chemotherapy-induced nausea and vomiting. J Clin Oncol 2005;23(28):7188–98.

[45] Stjernsward J, Colleau SM, Ventafridda V. The World Health Organization Cancer Pain and Palliative Care Program. Past, present, and future. J Pain Symptom Manage 1996; 12(2):65–72.

[46] van den Beuken-van Everdingen MH, de Rijke JM, Kessels AG, et al. Prevalence of pain in patients with cancer: a systematic review of the past 40 years. Ann Oncol 2007;18(9): 1437–49.

[47] Reid CM, Gooberman-Hill R, Hanks GW. Opioid analgesics for cancer pain: symptom control for the living or comfort for the dying? A qualitative study to investigate the factors influencing the decision to accept morphine for pain caused by cancer. Ann Oncol 2008;19(1):44–8.

[48] Villars P, Dodd M, West C, et al. Differences in the prevalence and severity of side effects based on type of analgesic prescription in patients with chronic cancer pain. J Pain Symptom Manage 2007;33(1):67–77.

[49] Kwon YD, Pittler MH, Ernst E. Acupuncture for peripheral joint osteoarthritis: a systematic review and meta-analysis. Rheumatology (Oxford) 2006;45(11):1331–7.

[50] White A, Foster NE, Cummings M, et al. Acupuncture treatment for chronic knee pain: a systematic review. Rheumatology (Oxford) 2007;46(3):384–90.

[51] Manheimer E, Linde K, Lao L, et al. Meta-analysis: acupuncture for osteoarthritis of the knee. Ann Intern Med 2007;146(12):868–77.

[52] Green S, Buchbinder R, Hetrick S. Acupuncture for shoulder pain. Cochrane Database Syst Rev 2005;(2):CD005319.

[53] Trinh K, Graham N, Gross A, et al. Acupuncture for neck disorders. Spine 2007;32(2): 236–43.

[54] Ernst E, Pittler MH. The effectiveness of acupuncture in treating acute dental pain: a systematic review. Br Dent J 1998;184(9):443–7.

[55] Clark D. Total pain, disciplinary power and the body in the work of Cicely Saunders, 1958–1967. Soc Sci Med 1999;49(6):727–36.

[56] Kaptchuk TJ, Stason WB, Davis RB, et al. Sham device v inert pill: randomised controlled trial of two placebo treatments. BMJ 2006;332(7538):391–7.

[57] Gejervall AL, Stener-Victorin E, Moller A, et al. Electro-acupuncture versus conventional analgesia: a comparison of pain levels during oocyte aspiration and patients' experiences of well-being after surgery. Hum Reprod 2005;20(3):728–35.

[58] Lin JG, Lo MW, Wen YR, et al. The effect of high- and low-frequency electro-acupuncture in pain after lower abdominal surgery. Pain 2002;99(3):509–14.

[59] Sim CK, Xu PC, Pua HL, et al. Effects of electro-acupuncture on intraoperative and postoperative analgesic requirement. Acupunct Med 2002;20(2–3):56–65.

[60] Usichenko TI, Dinse M, Hermsen M, et al. Auricular acupuncture for pain relief after total hip arthroplasty—a randomized controlled study. Pain 2005;114(3):320–7.

[61] Wong RH, Lee TW, Sihoe AD, et al. Analgesic effect of electro-acupuncture in post-thoracotomy pain: a prospective randomized trial. Ann Thorac Surg 2006;81(6): 2031–6.

[62] Mehling WE, Jacobs B, Acree M, et al. Symptom management with massage and acupuncture in postoperative cancer patients: a randomized controlled trial. J Pain Symptom Manage 2007;33(3):258–66.

[63] Chae Y, Yeom M, Han JH, et al. Effect of acupuncture on anxiety-like behavior during nicotine withdrawal and relevant mechanisms. Neurosci Lett 2008;430(2):98–102.

[64] Hansson Y, Carlsson C, Olsson E. Intramuscular and periosteal acupuncture for anxiety and sleep quality in patients with chronic musculoskeletal pain—an evaluator blind, controlled study. Acupunct Med 2007;25(4):148–57.

[65] Karst M, Winterhalter M, Munte S, et al. Auricular acupuncture for dental anxiety: a randomized controlled trial. Anesth Analg 2007;104(2):295–300.

[66] Spence DW, Kayumov L, Chen A, et al. Acupuncture increases nocturnal melatonin secretion and reduces insomnia and anxiety: a preliminary report. J Neuropsychiatry Clin Neurosci 2004;16(1):19–28.

[67] Wang SM, Kain ZN. Auricular acupuncture: a potential treatment for anxiety. Anesth Analg 2001;92(2):548–53.

[68] Wang SM, Peloquin C, Kain ZN. The use of auricular acupuncture to reduce preoperative anxiety. Anesth Analg 2001;93(5):1178–80, table of contents.

[69] Agarwal A, Ranjan R, Dhiraaj S, et al. Acupressure for prevention of preoperative anxiety: a prospective, randomised, placebo-controlled study. Anaesthesia 2005;60(10): 978–81.

[70] Kober A, Scheck T, Schubert B, et al. Auricular acupressure as a treatment for anxiety in prehospital transport settings. Anesthesiology 2003;98(6):1328–32.

[71] Mora B, Iannuzzi M, Lang T, et al. Auricular acupressure as a treatment for anxiety before extracorporeal shock wave lithotripsy in the elderly. J Urol 2007;178(1):160–4 [discussion: 164].

[72] Walker G, de Valois B, Davies R, et al. Ear acupuncture for hot flushes—the perceptions of women with breast cancer. Complement Ther Clin Pract 2007;13(4):250–7.

[73] Deng G, Vickers A, Yeung S, et al. Randomized, controlled trial of acupuncture for the treatment of hot flashes in breast cancer patients. J Clin Oncol 2007;25(35): 5584–90.

[74] Nedstrand E, Wyon Y, Hammar M, et al. Psychological well-being improves in women with breast cancer after treatment with applied relaxation or electro-acupuncture for vasomotor symptom. J Psychosom Obstet Gynaecol 2006;27(4):193–9.

[75] Chen C, Zhang Z, Li H, et al. Electro-acupuncture on Zusangli (ST36) to reduce chemotherapy-induced toxicity. Xin Zhong Yi (New Journal of Traditional Chinese Medicine) 2004;36(3):46–7.

[76] Du X, Gou Y, Chen F, et al. Compare different timing acupuncture on mitigating blood impairment caused by chemotherapy. Chinese Acupuncture Moxibustion 1994;14(3): 113–5.

[77] Li Y, Yu Y, Dai T. Clinical study on acupuncture treating side effects of radiation–chemotherapy with malignant tumours. Chinese Acupuncture Moxibustion 1997;17(6):327–8.

[78] Lu W, Matulonis UA, Doherty-Gilman A, et al. Acupuncture for chemotherapy-induced neutropenia in patients with gynecologic malignancies: a pilot randomized, sham-controlled clinical trial. Presented at: Society for Integrative Oncology 4th Annual Conference. San Francisco, November 15–17, 2007.

[79] Lu W, Metulonis UA, Doherty-Gilman A, et al. Granulocyte colony-stimulating factor (G-CSF) levels in a randomized, controlled acupuncture trial for chemotherapy-induced neutropenia. ASH Annual Meeting Abstracts 2007;110(11):4088.

[80] Molassiotis A, Sylt P, Diggins H. The management of cancer-related fatigue after chemotherapy with acupuncture and acupressure: a randomised controlled trial. Complement Ther Med 2007;15(4):228–37.

[81] Wong R, Sagar S. Acupuncture treatment for chemotherapy-induced peripheral neuropathy—a case series. Acupunct Med 2006;24(2):87–91.

[82] Chen HY, Shi Y, Ng CS, et al. Auricular acupuncture treatment for insomnia: a systematic review. J Altern Complement Med 2007;13(6):669–76.

[83] Cheuk DK, Yeung WF, Chung KF, et al. Acupuncture for insomnia. Cochrane Database Syst Rev 2007;(3):CD005472.

[84] Blom M, Dawidson I, Angmar-Mansson B. The effect of acupuncture on salivary flow rates in patients with xerostomia. Oral Surg Oral Med Oral Pathol 1992;73(3):293–8.

[85] Blom M, Lundeberg T. Long-term follow-up of patients treated with acupuncture for xerostomia and the influence of additional treatment. Oral Dis 2000;6(1):15–24.

[86] Johnstone PA, Niemtzow RC, Riffenburgh RH. Acupuncture for xerostomia: clinical update. Cancer 2002;94(4):1151–6.

[87] Maa SH, Sun MF, Hsu KH, et al. Effect of acupuncture or acupressure on quality of life of patients with chronic obstructive asthma: a pilot study. J Altern Complement Med 2003;9(5):659–70.

[88] Maa SH, Tsou TS, Wang KY, et al. Self-administered acupressure reduces the symptoms that limit daily activities in bronchiectasis patients: pilot study findings. J Clin Nurs 2007;16(4):794–804.

[89] Wu HS, Wu SC, Lin JG, et al. Effectiveness of acupressure in improving dyspnoea in chronic obstructive pulmonary disease. J Adv Nurs 2004;45(3):252–9.

[90] Dean-Clower E, Doherty-Gilman A, Rosenthal DS. The effect of acupuncture on the pain, nausea, and quality of life of patients with advanced cancer. Presented at the Society for Integrative Oncology 1st International Conference New York, NY, November 17–19, 2004.

[91] MacPherson H, Thomas K, Walters S, et al. The York acupuncture safety study: prospective survey of 34,000 treatments by traditional acupuncturists. BMJ 2001;323(7311):486–7.

[92] Weiger WA, Smith M, Boon H, et al. Advising patients who seek complementary and alternative medical therapies for cancer. Ann Intern Med 2002;137(11):889–903.

[93] FDA. Acupuncture needle status changed. Available at: http://www.fda.gov/bbs/topics/answers/ans00722.html. Accessed January 25, 2008.

[94] Burstein HJ, Gelber S, Guadagnoli E, et al. Use of alternative medicine by women with early stage breast cancer. N Engl J Med 1999;340(22):1733–9.

[95] Ganz PA, Desmond KA, Leedham B, et al. Quality of life in long-term, disease-free survivors of breast cancer: a follow-up study. J Natl Cancer Inst 2002;94(1):39–49.

[96] Vickers AJ. Can acupuncture have specific effects on health? A systematic review of acupuncture antiemesis trials. J R Soc Med 1996;89(6):303–11.

[97] Schulz KF, Chalmers I, Hayes RJ, et al. Empirical evidence of bias. Dimensions of methodological quality associated with estimates of treatment effects in controlled trials. JAMA 1995;273(5):408–12.

[98] Lund I, Lundeberg T. Are minimal, superficial, or sham acupuncture procedures acceptable as inert placebo controls? Acupunct Med 2006;24(1):13–5.

[99] Lundeberg T, Lund I. Are reviews based on sham acupuncture procedures in fibromyalgia syndrome (FMS) valid? Acupunct Med 2007;25(3):100–6.

[100] McManus CA, Schnyer RN, Kong J, et al. Sham acupuncture devices—practical advice for researchers. Acupunct Med 2007;25(1–2):36–40.

[101] Streitberger K, Kleinhenz J. Introducing a placebo needle into acupuncture research. Lancet 1998;352(9125):364–5.
[102] Kong J, Gollub RL, Rosman IS, et al. Brain activity associated with expectancy-enhanced placebo analgesia as measured by functional magnetic resonance imaging. J Neurosci 2006;26(2):381–8.
[103] MacPherson H, White A, Cummings M, et al. Standards for reporting interventions in controlled trials of acupuncture: the STRICTA recommendations. Complement Ther Med 2001;9(4):246–9.

Hematol Oncol Clin N Am 22 (2008) 649–660

HEMATOLOGY/ONCOLOGY CLINICS
OF NORTH AMERICA

The Value of Massage Therapy in Cancer Care

Cynthia D. Myers, PhD, LMT, NCTMB[a,*],
Tracy Walton, LMT, MS[b], Brent J. Small, PhD[c]

[a]Integrative Medicine, Health Outcomes and Behavior Program, Moffitt Cancer Center, 12902 Magnolia Drive, MRC-PSY, Tampa, FL 33612, USA
[b]Training and Consultation: Caring for Clients with Cancer, 10 Sargent Street, Cambridge, MA 02140, USA
[c]Health Outcomes and Behavior Program, Moffitt Cancer Center, 12902 Magnolia Drive, MRC-PSY, Tampa, FL 33612, USA

Massage therapy is increasingly being made available to patients in medical centers in North America as a supportive therapy to enhance comfort and help manage symptoms and side effects before, during, and after cancer treatment. Increased availability of massage to cancer patients results from several factors. Foremost is evidence of benefit of massage to cancer patients for symptom management in most studies conducted on this topic over the past two decades [1–24]. Citing this research and their own experiences and observations, massage therapists, patients, nurses, and others have advocated for inclusion of massage therapy in medical settings. Massage educators have authored texts [25,26], articles [27,28], and coursework materials to guide massage therapists in the myriad of factors informing sound clinical judgment regarding massage practice in the context of cancer treatment, producing a cohort of oncology-trained massage therapists. Collectively, these factors contribute to the current climate in which oncology massage is recommended for cancer patients experiencing anxiety or pain [29], and oncology massage is becoming an established subspecialty of therapeutic massage. In 2007 the first national meeting of oncology massage professionals drew over 160 participants and faculty from across North America [30]. Out of this meeting, a new professional society was formed, the Society for Oncology Massage, which incorporated with the mission of linking cancer patients, their families, and caregivers with skilled oncology massage therapists [31].

There are many styles of massage therapy and hands-on soft tissue therapies. These therapies have in common the use of manual manipulation of soft tissue through contact, pressure, or movement with the intended purpose of

This article is supported by grant R21CA098408 from the National Cancer Institute.

*Corresponding author. E-mail address: cynthia.myers@moffitt.org (CD. Myers).

enhancing well-being. They differ widely in their theoretic bases, specific techniques, training, and regulatory requirements. Massage therapies studied with cancer patients have included Swedish massage, aromatherapy massage, reflexology, acupressure, and manual lymphatic drainage. In the context of cancer care, Swedish massage aims to reduce excess muscle tension and promote relaxation and comfort by providing broad, flowing, soothing strokes (effleurage) applied with lotion or massage oil, from distal to proximal on extremities, and gentle kneading of soft tissues (petrissage). Aromatherapy massage blends selected scented oils into massage oil with the idea that doing so enhances the beneficial effects of massage on physical and emotional well-being. Studies of reflexology for cancer patients have focused on manual pressure to specific areas of the feet theoretically linked with remote areas of the body with the goal of enhancing well-being. Acupressure massage derives from meridian theory of traditional Chinese medicine on which acupuncture is based, using focal pressure rather than penetration by acupuncture needles with the goal of adjusting the flow of life-force to promote health and manage symptoms. Manual lymphatic drainage applies light, flowing strokes in specific patterns with the goal of alleviating lymphedema. This article provides a summary of findings of peer-reviewed research on massage therapy showing beneficial effects associated with massage in terms of easing symptoms and side effects in cancer treatment.

METHODS OF RESEARCH LITERATURE REVIEW

The Cumulative Index to Nursing and Allied Health Literature and the National Library of Medicine PubMed databases were searched from their inception through 2007 to locate studies in which a self-report measure of at least one symptom or side effect was administered to patients before and after massage. Studies of combined approaches (eg, massage combined with acupuncture, manual lymphatic drainage combined with compression bandaging) were not included. Search terms were "massage," "effleurage," "petrissage," "reflexology," or "acupressure" paired with cancer.

RESULTS

Twenty-four studies were located in which at least one symptom or side effect was assessed by patient self-report before and after massage. Symptoms and side effects assessed as outcomes included anxiety, pain, nausea, depression, and fatigue. Twelve studies were located on Swedish massage [1–12], five studies on aromatherapy massage [13–17], five on reflexology [4,18–21], and three on acupressure [22–24]. The studies reporting beneficial effects associated with massage are summarized in Tables 1–4, which provide the author, study description, and findings for controlled between-group comparisons or, where no controlled results are available, for within-group (pre-post) comparisons. Alpha of less than 0.05 was chosen for statistical significance. Studies of manual lymphatic drainage found by the literature search emphasized volumetric outcomes of massage applied in conjunction with complete decongestive therapy rather than self-report of symptoms or side effects in relation only to massage; studies of manual lymphatic drainage are not discussed in this article.

With regard to measurement tools used to assess outcomes, most studies used standardized self-report questionnaires. Anxiety was assessed with numerical rating scales (NRS), visual analog scales (VAS), the Hospital Anxiety and Depression Scale [32], the Profile of Mood States [33], the State Trait Anxiety Inventory [34], the Symptom Checklist–90 Revised [35], the European Organization for Research and Treatment of Cancer Quality of Life Questionnaire (EORTC QLQ-C30) [36], and a shortened version of the Structured Clinical Interview [37]. Pain was assessed with NRS, VAS, the Brief Pain Inventory [38], the Memorial Pain Assessment Card [39], the McGill Pain Questionnaire Short-Form [40], and the EORTC QLQ-C30 [36]. Fatigue was assessed with NRS, VAS, and the EORTC QLQ-C30 [36]. Nausea was assessed with NRS; VAS; a brief nausea index used by Post-White and colleagues [8], based on a modification of the Brief Pain Inventory [38]; the Rhodes Inventory of Nausea, Vomiting, and Retching [41]; a chemotherapy problem checklist; and a daily log. Depression was assessed by NRS, VAS, the Beck Depression Inventory [42], the Hospital Anxiety and Depression Scale [32], the Profile of Mood States [33], the Symptom Checklist–90 Revised [35], and the Centers for Epidemiologic Studies–Depression scale [43].

Collectively, the available results, although not uniform, suggest beneficial effects associated with massage for many cancer patients, particularly with regard to helping with anxiety and pain. Massage therapy has previously been found reliably to reduce state anxiety in other patient and nonpatient samples in a meta-analysis [44]. Anxiety reduction is of clear clinical relevance to cancer patients, from the initial acute adjustment of receiving a cancer diagnosis; to the stress of awaiting further diagnostic test results; to anticipatory and concurrent anxiety in relation to treatment, side effects, and disruption of normal life and role functioning; to the prospect of facing real or potential disease recurrence [45]. A beneficial future direction for research is to study the integration of massage therapy into prevention and control of anxiety in cancer patients at increased risk of clinically significant anxiety, such as those with a premorbid history of elevated anxiety or experiencing higher levels of anxiety about cancer treatment [46].

Beneficial massage effects on pain were reported in several studies. Patient selection based on pain etiology, and detailed characterization of pain at baseline in future studies may clarify the effects of massage on pain, as compared with studies to date that have included heterogeneous patient samples. Etiology of cancer pain varies widely, such as bone pain caused by metastases, versus side effects or late effects of treatment, such as peripheral neuropathy, postsurgical pain, or postradiation pain. One massage style may potentially be more beneficial than another for a specific type of cancer pain. This is currently not known. Examination of the temporal pattern of massage effects on pain, including the possibility that improved sleep following massage, which is often reported by patients, may lead to better pain control, is a valuable area for future research.

Table 1
Studies showing benefit associated with Swedish massage provided to adult cancer patients

Reference	Patient sample	Design	Benefits associated with Swedish massage
Ahles et al [1]	Inpatient, mixed diagnoses, undergoing bone marrow transplant (N = 34)	Randomized, controlled. Group 1 = 4–9 20-min massages to shoulders, neck, face, scalp (N = 16) Group 2 = 20-min quiet time (N = 18)	Decreased anxiety, nausea
Billhult et al [2]	Women with breast cancer during outpatient chemotherapy (N = 39)	Randomized controlled. Group 1 = 5 20-min massages to foot/lower leg or hand/lower arm (N = 19) Group 2 = 5 20-min visits from hospital staff (N = 20)	Decreased nausea
Campeau et al [3]	Outpatient, mixed diagnosis, receiving radiation therapy (N = 100)	Randomized controlled. Group 1 = 10 15-min massages back, arms, hands, neck, scalp (N =52) Group 2 = usual care (N = 48)	Decreased anxiety
Cassileth and Vickers [4]	Inpatient and outpatient, mixed diagnosis (N = 560)	Observational uncontrolled. Average of 20 min for inpatients and 60 min for outpatients	Decreased pain, fatigue, anxiety, nausea, depression
Ferrell-Torry and Glick [5]	Inpatient males with pain, mixed diagnoses (N = 9)	Observational uncontrolled. 30 min massage to feet, back, neck, shoulders with deep breathing on two consecutive evenings	Decreased pain, anxiety
Grealish et al [6]	Inpatient, mixed diagnoses (32 metastatic) (N =87)	Subjects as own control randomized to order. 10-min foot massage 2 out of 3 consecutive evenings versus 10 min of quiet activity 1 of 3 days	Decreased pain, nausea

Study	Population	Design/intervention	Results
Hernandez-Reif et al [7]	Outpatient women early stage I–III breast cancer in past 3 y (N = 58)	Randomized controlled. Group 1 = 30-min full-body massage 3 times per week for 5 weeks (N = 22). Group 2 = 30-min progressive muscle relaxation audiotape 3 times per week for 5 wk (N= 20) Group 3 = Usual care (N = 16)	Decreased pain, anxiety, depression
Post-White et al [8]	Outpatient, mixed diagnoses from chemotherapy clinics, at least one symptom ≥3/10 (N = 164)	Controlled crossover mixed between/within design. Group 1 = 4 weekly 45-min full-body massages (N = 62). Group 2 = 4 weekly 45-min healing touch (N = 56). Group 3 = 4 weekly 45-min staff presence (n = 45). All versus 4 wk usual care.	Decreased pain, anxiety
Toth et al [10]	Inpatient, advanced cancer (N = 6, data on symptoms available for 4)	Observational uncontrolled. From 1 to 9 massages provided, 15–60 min (average, 34) in duration, in evenings	Decreased fatigue
Weinrich and Weinrich [11]	Inpatient, mixed diagnoses (N = 28)	Randomized controlled. Group 1 = 10-min back massage (N = 14) Group 2 = 10-min visit (N = 14)	Decreased pain
Wilkie et al [12]	Hospice patients, mixed diagnoses (N = 29)	Randomized controlled. Group 1 = 30–50 min full-body massage twice weekly for 2 wk (N = 15) Group 2 = usual hospice care (N = 14)	Decreased pain

Table 2
Studies showing benefit associated with aromatherapy massage provided to adult cancer patients

Reference	Patient sample	Design, intervention, and control	Benefits associated with aromatherapy massage
Corner et al [13]	Patients on active treatment, mixed diagnoses (N = 52)	Randomized, matched control. Group 1 = 8 weekly 30-min back massages with aromatherapy (N = 18). Group 2 = 8 weekly 30-min back massages with almond oil (N = 17). Group 3 = usual care (N = 18).	Decreased anxiety, depression
Soden et al [15]	Palliative care patients, mixed advanced cancer diagnoses (N = 42)	Randomized controlled. Group 1 = 4 weekly 30-min back massage with lavender/sweet almond oil (N = 16). Group 2 = 4 weekly 30-min back massage with sweet almond oil (N = 13).Control = usual care (N = 13)	Decreased pain
Wilkinson et al [17]	Outpatient and palliative patients, mixed diagnoses (N = 288)	Randomized controlled. Group 1 = 4 weekly 60-min massage with blends of 20 essential oils (N = 144). Control = usual care (N = 144)	Decreased anxiety

Table 3
Studies showing benefit associated with reflexology provided to adult cancer patients

Reference	Patient sample	Design	Benefits associated with reflexology
Cassileth and Vickers [4]	Inpatient and outpatient, mixed diagnoses (N = 585)	Observational uncontrolled Reflexology foot massage average of 20 min for inpatients and 60 min for outpatients	Decreased pain, fatigue, anxiety, nausea, and depression
Quattrin et al [18]	Inpatient receiving chemotherapy, mixed diagnoses (N = 30)	Controlled. Quasi-experimental (not randomized). Group 1 = 30-min foot reflexology session (N = 15). Control = usual care (N = 15)	Decreased pain, anxiety
Stephenson et al [21]	Inpatient with breast or lung cancer reporting anxiety (N = 23)	Self as own control, crossover design. 30-min reflexology versus 30-min period of time at least 48 h postreflexology	Decreased pain, anxiety
Stephenson et al [20]	Inpatient with metastatic cancer, mixed diagnoses, reporting pain (N = 36)	Randomized controlled Group 1 = 2 sessions of foot reflexology 24 hours apart (N = 19) Group 2 = usual care (N = 17)	Decreased pain

Table 4
Studies showing benefit associated with acupressure provided to adult cancer patients

References	Patient sample	Design, intervention, and control	Benefits associated with acupressure
Dibble et al [22]	Outpatient women receiving chemotherapy for breast cancer (N = 17)	Randomized controlled. Group 1 = manually self-administered acupressure at P6 or ST36 points daily for maximum 3 min plus as needed (N = 8) Group 2 = usual care (N = 9)	Decreased nausea
Dibble et al [23]	Women beginning second or third cycle of chemotherapy for breast cancer, with moderate nausea on previous chemotherapy cycle (N = 160).	Randomized controlled. Group 1 = 3 min self-administered acupressure per arm at P6 point each morning and as needed during the day for nausea (N = 53). Group 2 = 3 min self-administered acupressure per hand at placebo acupressure point and as needed during the day for nausea (N = 53) Group 3 = usual care (N = 54)	Decreased delayed nausea and vomiting
Shin et al [24]	Inpatient gastric cancer (N = 40)	Controlled, not random assignment (first 20 assigned usual care, next 20 assigned acupressure). Group 1 = 5 min of acupressure at P6 point before chemotherapy and mealtimes, and anytime nausea was felt (N = 20) Group 2 = usual care (N = 20)	Decreased nausea

Methodologic weaknesses of many of the studies, such as small sample sizes, are noted. For example, blinding of massage therapists, data collectors, or participants has been inconsistent, and could be strengthened in future studies by keeping the experimental hypothesis from these parties. Assessing pretreatment and posttreatment credibility of interventions and expectancies of participants, data collectors, and massage therapists could also prove helpful [47]. Most studies provided no rationale for the number or length of massages provided. Unlike pharmaceutical studies where a dose finding phase is required, no such systematic approach is taken to determining the optimal dose of massage before implementing a trial. Ideally, this would be a helpful aspect to pilot before launching future large-scale studies targeting specific outcomes.

Within-group comparisons of symptoms before and after massage have often produced more impressive improvements than controlled comparisons. Attribution of symptom reduction to massage in uncontrolled studies may be inaccurate, because nonspecific factors of the intervention (eg, attention), the passage of time, or regression to the mean may explain observed improvements. Appropriate control groups for massage studies are challenging to construct and are the subject of debate and discussion [44,48,49]. Smith and colleagues [48] have provided an instructive, in-depth discussion of the process they used to select control and comparison groups when designing the largest National Institutes of Health–funded randomized trial to date on oncology massage. Control groups must be dictated by the research aims, whether that is to demonstrate additional benefit over usual care, or to isolate specific effective elements of massage. Replication of study findings by different investigators is needed to establish efficacy.

No serious adverse events were reported in any of the studies; however, in most studies it is not clear that data were collected on mild or adverse events, either acute or delayed. Most studies report only the immediate effects of massage. Data are needed on the effects of massage over the hours and days following massage sessions. To illustrate, clinical experience indicates that some patients report beneficial effects of full-body massage received in the hours after chemotherapy infusion [25], whereas others have attributed flulike symptoms to full-body massage received within a day of chemotherapy and recommend against this option [50]. Prevalence and predictors of these opposite outcomes are currently unknown.

This article is limited to massage effects on symptoms and side effects reported by adult cancer patients, and is not a comprehensive review of all literature on massage for cancer patients. Other studies have reported on the impact of massage on quality of life and on objective outcomes, such as lymphedema, respiration rate, blood pressure, cortisol levels, and time to engraftment following bone marrow transplantation. Included are only manually administered massage, and not review papers on acupressure massage using mechanical stimulation of acupressure points [51]. The important topic of the core competencies of oncology-trained massage therapists is beyond the scope of this article, and has been addressed elsewhere, along with information about training programs in oncology massage [52]. Training of family members to provide safe, gentle, supportive massage is also an important area of active research, early results of which suggest feasibility of such training and beneficial and cost-effective results to patients and family members [53–55]. Finally, additional studies are needed on massage provided to children and young patients with cancer to determine the potential benefits of massage to them for reducing symptoms and side effects.

SUMMARY

Massage therapy is offered at several major cancer centers in North America. Two decades of data point to benefits of gentle massage when properly modified. Future studies should attempt to replicate and extend preliminary studies using rigorous study designs, adequate statistical power, assessment of potential adverse effects, identification of predictors of response to massage, and psychologic and biologic mechanisms of massage. Evidence-based massage provided by properly trained individuals can provide a soothing and nurturing experience in the midst of stressful cancer treatment, and it should be made available to patients to assist in the optimal prevention and control of cancer symptoms and treatment side effects.

References

[1] Ahles TA, Tope DM, Pinkson B, et al. Massage therapy for patients undergoing autologous bone marrow transplantation. J Pain Symptom Manage 1999;18(3):157–63.

[2] Billhult A, Bergbom I, Stener-Victorin E. Massage relieves nausea in women with breast cancer who are undergoing chemotherapy. J Altern Complement Med 2007;13(1):53–7.

[3] Campeau M-P, Gaboriault R, Drapeau M, et al. Impact of massage therapy on anxiety levels in patients undergoing radiation therapy: randomized controlled trial. J Soc Integr Oncol 2007;5(4):133–8.

[4] Cassileth B, Vickers AJ. Massage therapy for symptom control: outcome study at a major cancer center. J Pain Symptom Manage 2004;28(3):244–9.

[5] Ferrell-Torry AT, Glick OJ. The use of therapeutic massage as a nursing intervention to modify anxiety and the perception of cancer pain. Cancer Nurs 1993;16(2):93–101.

[6] Grealish L, Lomasney A, Whiteman B. Foot massage: a nursing intervention to modify the distressing symptoms of pain and nausea in patients hospitalized with cancer. Cancer Nurs 2000;23(3):237–43.

[7] Hernandez-Reif M, Field T, Ironson G, et al. Natural killer cells and lymphocytes increase in women with breast cancer following massage therapy. Int J Neurosci 2005;115(4):495–510.

[8] Post-White J, Kinney ME, Savik KS, et al. Therapeutic massage and healing touch improve symptoms in cancer. Integr Cancer Ther 2003;2(4):332–44.

[9] Smith MC, Kemp J, Hemphill L, et al. Outcomes of therapeutic massage for hospitalized cancer patients. J Nurs Scholarsh 2002;34(3):257–62.

[10] Toth M, Kahn J, Walton T, et al. Therapeutic massage intervention for hospitalized patients with cancer. Alternative and Complementary Therapies June 2003;1:17–24.

[11] Weinrich SP, Weinrich MC. The effect of massage on pain in cancer patients. Appl Nurs Res 1990;3:140–5.

[12] Wilkie DJ, Kampbell J, Cutshall S, et al. Effects of massage on pain intensity, analgesics and quality of life in patients with cancer pain: a pilot study of a randomized clinical trial conducted within hospice care delivery. Hosp J 2000;15(3):31–53.

[13] Corner J, Cawley N, Hildebrand S. An evaluation of the use of massage and essential oils on the wellbeing of cancer patients. Int J Palliat Nurs 1995;1(2):67–73.

[14] Hadfield N. The role of aromatherapy massage in reducing anxiety in patients with malignant brain tumours. Int J Palliat Nurs 2001;7(6):279–85.

[15] Soden K, Vincent K, Craske S, et al. A randomized controlled trial of aromatherapy massage in a hospice setting. Palliat Med 2004;18:87–92.

[16] Wilkinson S, Aldridge J, Salmon I, et al. An evaluation of aromatherapy massage in palliative care. Palliat Med 1999;13:409–17.

[17] Wilkinson SM, Love SB, Westcombe AM, et al. Effectiveness of aromatherapy massage in the management of anxiety and depression in patients with cancer: a multicenter randomized controlled trial. J Clin Oncol 2007;25(5):532–9.

[18] Quattrin R, Zanini A, Buchini S, et al. Use of reflexology foot massage to reduce anxiety in hospitalized cancer patients in chemotherapy treatment: methodology and outcomes. J Nurs Manag 2006;14(2):96–105.

[19] Ross CSK, Hamilton J, Macrae G, et al. A pilot study to evaluate the effect of reflexology on mood and symptom rating of advanced cancer patients. Palliat Med 2002;16:544–5.

[20] Stephenson N, Dalton JA, Carlson J. The effect of foot reflexology on pain in patients with metastatic cancer. Appl Nurs Res 2003;16(4):284–6.

[21] Stephenson NL, Weinrich SP, Tavakoli AS. The effects of foot reflexology on anxiety and pain in patients with breast and lung cancer. Oncol Nurs Forum 2000;27(1):67–72.

[22] Dibble SL, Chapman J, Mack KA, et al. Acupressure for nausea: results of a pilot study. Oncol Nurs Forum 2000;27(1):1–12.

[23] Dibble SL, Luce J, Cooper BA, et al. Acupressure for chemotherapy-induced nausea and vomiting: a randomized clinical trial. Oncol Nurs Forum 2007;34(4):813–20.

[24] Shin YH, Kim TI, Shin MS, et al. Effect of acupressure on nausea and vomiting during chemotherapy cycle for Korean postoperative stomach cancer patients. Cancer Nurs 2004;27(4):267–74.

[25] MacDonald G. Medicine hands: massage therapy for people with cancer. Findhorn (Scotland): Findhorn Press; 1999 [revised edition 2007].

[26] Curties D. Massage therapy and cancer. Moncton (NB): Curties-Overzet Publications; 1999.

[27] Walton T. Cancer and massage therapy: essential contraindications. Massage Therapy Journal 2006;45(2):119–34. Available at: http://www.amtamassage.org/journal/archived_issues.html. Accessed Feb 5, 2008.

[28] Walton T. Cancer and massage therapy: contraindications and cancer treatment. Massage Therapy Journal 2006;45(3):119–34. Available at: http://www.amtamassage.org/journal/archived_issues.html. Accessed Feb 5, 2008.

[29] Deng GE, Cassileth BR, Cohen L, et al. Integrative oncology practice guidelines. J Soc Integr Oncol 2007;5(2):65–84.

[30] Oncology Massage Healing Summit. Available at: http://www.mercycollege.edu/oncology_conf.php. Accessed Feb 5, 2008.

[31] Society for Oncology Massage. Available at: http://www.s4om.org/. Accessed Feb 5, 2008.

[32] Zigmond AS, Snaith RP. The hospital anxiety and depression scale. Acta Psychiatr Scand 1983;67(6):361–70.

[33] McNair D, Lorr M, Droppleman L. Profile of mood states. San Diego (CA): Education and Industrial Testing Service; 1992.

[34] Spielberger C, Gorsuch R, Lushene R. Manual for the state-trait anxiety inventory. Palo Alto (CA): Consulting Psychologist Press; 1970.

[35] Derogatis L. Administration, scoring, and procedural manual II. Towson (MD): Clinical Psychometric Research; 1993.

[36] Fayers P, Aaronson N, Bjordal K, et al. EORTC QLQ-C30 Scoring Manual. 3rd edition. Brussels (Belgium): European Organisation for Research and Treatment of Cancer; 2001.

[37] First MB, Spitzer RL, Gibbon M, et al. Structured clinical interview for DSM Axis I disorders. Arlington (VA): American Psychiatric Publishing, Inc.; 1997.

[38] Daut RL, Cleeland CS, Flanery RC. Development of the Wisconsin Brief Pain Questionnaire to assess pain in cancer and other diseases. Pain 1983;17:197–210.

[39] Fishman B, Pasternak S, Wallenstein SL, et al. The Memorial Pain Assessment Card: a valid instrument for the evaluation of cancer pain. Cancer 1987;60(5):1151–8.

[40] Melzack R. The short-form McGill Pain Questionnaire. Pain 1987;30(2):191–7.

[41] Rhodes VA, Watson PM, Johnson MH. Development of reliable and valid measures of nausea and vomiting. Cancer Nurs 1984;7(1):33–41.

[42] Beck AT, Ward CH, Mendelson M, et al. An inventory for measuring depression. Arch Gen Psychiatry 1961;4:561–71.

[43] Radloff L. The CES-D scale: a self report depression scale for research in the general population. Applied Psychosocial Measurement 1977;1:384–401.

[44] Moyer CA, Rounds J, Hannum JW. A meta-analysis of massage therapy research. Psychol Bull 2004;130(1):3–18.

[45] Stark D, Kiely M, Smith A, et al. Anxiety disorders in cancer patients: their nature, associations, and relation to quality of life. J Clin Oncol 2002;20(14):3137–48.

[46] Breitbart W. Identifying patients at risk for, and treatment of major psychiatric complications of cancer. Support Care Cancer 1995;3(1):45–60.

[47] Mehling W, DiBlasi Z, Hecht F. Bias control in trials of bodywork: a review of methodological issues. J Altern Complement Med 2005;11(2):333–42.

[48] Smith M, Kutner J, Hemphill L, et al. Developing treatment and control conditions in a clinical trial of massage therapy for advanced cancer. J Soc Integr Oncol 2007;5(4):139–46.

[49] Ezzo J. What can be learned from Cochrane systematic reviews of massage that can guide future research? J Altern Complement Med 2007;13(2):291–5.

[50] Versagi CM. Cancer and massage therapy: is your therapist trained to meet your needs? Women and Cancer Spring 2007;84–8.

[51] Ezzo JM, Richardson MA, Vickers A, et al. Acupuncture-point stimulation for chemotherapy-induced nausea or vomiting (review). Cochrane Database Syst Rev 2006;19(2):CD002285.

[52] Miner W. Training massage therapists to work in oncology. J Soc Integr Oncol 2007;5(4): 163–6.

[53] Collinge W, Kahn J, Yarnold P, et al. Couples and cancer: feasibility of brief instruction in massage and touch therapy to build caregiver efficacy. J Soc Integr Oncol 2007;5(4): 147–54.

[54] Myers C, Yokum D, Wilson J, et al. Family-administered massage for young patients with cancer. J Soc Integr Oncol 2007;5(4):181 [abstract].

[55] Stephenson NL, Swanson M, Dalton J, et al. Partner-delivered reflexology: effects on cancer pain and anxiety. Oncol Nurs Forum 2007;34(1):127–32.

Hematol Oncol Clin N Am 22 (2008) 661–670

HEMATOLOGY/ONCOLOGY CLINICS
OF NORTH AMERICA

Evidence-Based Botanical Research: Applications and Challenges

K. Simon Yeung, PharmD, LAc, Jyothirmai Gubili, MS*,
Barrie Cassileth, MS, PhD

Integrative Medicine Service, Memorial Sloan-Kettering Cancer Center, 1429 First Avenue,
New York, NY 10021, USA

The use of herbal supplements has grown significantly over the last three decades in the United States. According to a recent survey, nearly 20% Americans use botanicals [1]. Many cancer patients also use supplements in hopes of cure and for control of symptoms that often are controlled poorly with conventional medicine [2]. An estimated 13% to 63% of cancer patients use herbal supplements as adjuvant during and after chemotherapy [3]. Patients cite symptom control, quality-of-life issues, and cancer recurrence as major reasons for using these products [2,4,5]. Most herbal supplements, however, are marketed based on their traditional uses. Only limited data exist on the safety and efficacy of many botanicals because of paucity of research. This article discusses the unique applications and challenges in evidence-based botanical research, especially in the oncology setting.

In commerce, botanicals refer to products derived from plants, algae, and macroscopic fungi (even though fungi are not in the plant kingdom). They can be considered food when consumed for their nutrition value, taste, or aroma. This article focuses on botanical products that are used as dietary supplements to affect structure or function or as drugs to prevent or treat diseases. These also are referred to as herbal medicine or herbs. Use of botanicals falls under "biologically based practices" in the context of complementary and alternative medicine by the National Center for Complementary and Alternative Medicine (NCCAM).

Botanical products used in research can be raw herbs (whole or cut plants or isolated plant parts); herbal materials (processed herbs, juices, resins, or oils); or herbal preparations (purified or extracted components mixed with other materials). The finished products may contain multiple ingredients and may take the form of powder, liquid, pills, or topical preparations. Most herbs have long history of use for specific diseases in traditional medicine. Some existing herbs, however, are investigated for new uses, and there are studies on botanicals for novel indications that are not used commonly as food or drugs.

*Corresponding author. E-mail address: gubilij@mskcc.org (J. Gubili).

0889-8588/08/$ – see front matter
doi:10.1016/j.hoc.2008.04.007

WHY STUDY BOTANICALS?

To Validate Traditional Uses and Efficacy

Botanicals have been the source of medicine since the dawn of civilization and remain used by most people in the world, either as medicine in developing countries or as dietary supplements in numerous developed nations. Although herbs are associated with certain functions or indicated as treatment for diseases, the mechanisms of action of many herbs have not been elucidated fully, and the optimal doses are often unclear.

To Examine Safety

Although botanicals have been used for generations without incidents of adverse effects, long-term use is not proof of safety. Botanicals contain biologically active compounds that can cause adverse reactions and interact with new prescription medications [6,7]. For example, the popular herb St. John's wort (*Hypericum perforatum*) is used to treat depression [8], but it also induces cytochrome P450 3A4, an enzyme responsible for metabolism of many drugs, including those used during chemotherapy [9]. Botanicals research can provide useful information to patients and health care professionals to make educated decisions.

For Drug Development

Many drugs used in mainstream medicine are derived from plants. These include commonly used chemotherapy agents, like taxanes from Pacific yew (*Taxus brevifolia*) and vinca alkaloid from Madagascar periwinkle (*Catharanthus roseus*). There remain large numbers of flora, however, that have not been investigated, and they continue to be the source of novel drugs.

To Document Efficacy

Evidence-based research is required to provide scientific proof of safety and efficacy of botanical products. The following steps are essential for designing an effective study. The critical sequence of investigation is detailed.

EVIDENCE-BASED BOTANICAL RESEARCH

Literature Search

The first step is to review existing literature to provide the basis and justification for further studies. Botanicals that have been in general use for long periods of time may or may not be supported by some scientific evidence. Studies, however, often are limited to in vitro and animal studies, case reports, or small scale, poorly designed trials. Many are published in foreign language journals and must be translated into English. The culture of publishing only positive results and the unsophisticated peer review process in some countries casts doubts on the credibility of many of these publications, and they cannot be regarded as reliable.

Well-designed studies, however, have been published in the last decade and increasingly are followed by high-quality systematic reviews and meta-analyses in the Cochrane Collaboration database. Standard pharmacopeias now include monographs on selected botanicals. For example, the English version of the Chinese pharmacopeia has information on hundreds of Chinese medicinal herbs [10]. The German Commission E monographs contain information on the safety and efficacy of hundreds on botanicals [11].

Screening

The standard approach to drug discovery involves screening large numbers of botanicals or other agents using in vitro and animal models. Today computers that can be used to simulate molecular and bioactivity modeling by means of in silico studies are assisting these processes [12]. Botanicals that demonstrate the intended bioactivities are fractionated further. Active compounds are isolated to elucidate mechanism of action. They can be modified chemically to change or enhance the pharmacologic properties. Promising agents then are studied for toxicity, bioavailability, and gene expression following which, well-characterized and purified compounds will be tested in clinical trials. Only one in thousands of the original candidates eventually is approved and marketed as a drug.

The Drug Development Program, DTP, of the National Cancer Institute (NCI)/National Institutes of Health (NIH) maintains a Natural Products Repository that has over 50,000 plant samples from around the world through contracts with major botanical gardens and arboretums [13]. Information on botanical compounds screening is available to the public to facilitate further research [14].

Ethnobotany Approach

Although screening a large number of agents remains a time-proven method for drug discovery, researchers also use ethnobotany to aid in selecting useful botanicals [15]. The study of how different cultures or civilizations use local plants can yield valuable clues about their medicinal properties. Practitioners who have this knowledge, however, are usually shamans or native healers who administer herbs based on faith and spiritual beliefs. Training is usually through apprenticeship, and there is no standard method to identify medicinal plants. To use ethnobotany, researchers must work with ethnobotanists who have a thorough understanding of native culture and language. Researchers also need to respect the rights of indigenous people who may claim ownership to the study agents. They also have a moral obligation to make sure the local people benefit from the research.

DESIGNING BOTANICAL STUDIES

Modern biomedical research is hypothesis-driven. It is designed to answer specific research questions, such as whether a single chemical can be used to treat an isolated symptom or a disease. Traditional medicine, however, tends to use multiple herbs and treatment modalities to address disease. Often the paradigms are difficult to relate to standard research language. This raises questions about the wisdom of applying modern research methodology to traditional medicine and botanicals research. Some propose to study traditional medicine as a whole. This is sometimes referred to as a black box design [16], and allows practitioners to use traditional theories and methods to treat patients in a trial. Trained herbalists can custom-formulate botanical formulas to each individual's unique condition. Such an approach, however, results in multiple variables, too many to control in a scientific study. It also yields outcomes that are too broad to draw meaningful conclusions and therefore has limited scientific value.

Clinical Trials

Three-phase clinical studies using a single herbal ingredient or a predefined formula remain the norm, but designing a trial with an anticancer botanical incurs special challenges. First, history of use generally is employed to justify the safety of botanicals, but this does not indicate the safety of the product when used with pharmaceuticals in cancer treatment. Evidence of safety should include endpoints related to interactions with other drugs that could be used in combination.

As for dosage, historic or traditional dosage range typically is applied as the therapeutic dose. It is rare that a botanical treatment dose is determined according to results of a dose escalation trial. Such trials are important, especially when botanicals are used for their immunomodulating activities. These products usually have very low toxicity, and the traditional endpoint, the maximum tolerated dose (MTD) may not apply. Also, the dose curve may peak in a nonlinear fashion, indicating that higher dose may be less effective than a lower dose [17]. Therefore it is prudent to determine the safety and optimal dose in a phase 1 study. Innovative study methods have been developed to address the special characteristics of anticancer botanicals [18].

In phase 2 studies, botanical agents are administered to a larger group of people to check effectiveness and to further evaluate safety.

Phase 3 trials are conducted in large groups of people to confirm the effectiveness of the botanical, monitor its adverse effects, and compare it to commonly used treatments. Because of the complexity and high cost, only a handful of unpatented botanical products truly reach this level of research.

The inclusion of a placebo in clinical trials has generated much controversy in cancer research [19]. Many argue that a botanical product that is better than placebo is not good enough to be recommended for general use; it should be compared with a proven anticancer pharmaceutical. Others believe it is unethical to deny proven treatment for patients randomized in the placebo control group. Currently, placebos are no longer acceptable in cancer treatment trials. Using best existing care or botanicals in addition to standard treatment as control groups or a cross-over study are other options. Placebos, however, still are considered robust controls in botanicals trials for other indications, such as those used as immune enhancers. When a placebo is employed, inert coloring and flavoring agents are used to give it a final appearance similar to the study product to ensure blinding. Many herbs, however, have distinctive smell, taste, and texture that are hard to copy. Use of capsule dosage form can help to mask some of the differences. This has been applied successfully in previous trials [20,21].

ADDITIONAL CHALLENGES IN BOTANICALS RESEARCH

Although the methods and approaches used for botanicals research should replicate those applied in other disciplines, some challenges are unique to botanicals research.

Obtaining Botanicals

A major obstacle with botanical research is procuring appropriate materials for study. The study agent may be a single plant that requires collection and processing, or a commercially available product. Plants may be collected in the wild or cultivated. Those collected in the wild must be sorted and identified by trained personnel. The quantity may be limited, and future batches may be difficult to obtain, not entirely consistent with previous batches, or unavailable. The plant could be an endangered species or threatened by overharvesting. In the United States, if plants are collected in their native habitat, even in privately owned land, an environmental assessment (EA) may be required.

Botanicals marketed as dietary supplements generally are cultivated. These plants typically and optimally should be grown and collected in farms using good agricultural practices (GAP) and good handling practices (GHP) defined by the US Department of Agriculture (USDA) [22]. The United Nations and the European Union also have published similar guidelines [23]. Other countries may apply different standards. Specimens obtained this way are more reliable, as the source is known and future supply is ensured.

Importing Botanicals

To widen the scope of selection, it may be necessary to resort to native flora from abroad.

Shipping of plant materials for study in the United States can be a complicated process. Clearance may be needed from the exporting country. Some countries limit exportation of botanical products unless they meet certain requirements of product integrity. Importation of botanical products is under the scrutiny of many United States agencies in addition to the US Customs Office. A botanical imported for research may be considered a drug by the US Food and Drug Administration unless it already is marketed as a food product or a dietary supplement. Transportation of an unapproved drug requires filing an Investigational New Drug (IND) application. Additional information about the manufacturing and storage facilities must be provided under the new Bioterrorism Act. Recently, the FDA also issued regulation on current good manufacturing practices (cGMP) to ensure the quality of dietary supplements [24].

If the imported product falls under the Convention on International Trade in Endangered Species of Wild Fauna and Flora (CITES) Act or the Endangered Species Act (ESA), special permits maybe required from the US Department of Agriculture's Animal and Plant Health Inspection Service. This permits small samples of prohibited plants or plant products to be imported for experimental purposes. Shipments that contain live plants or seeds also are subjected to Phytosanitary Certification and additional inspections.

International carriers such as United Parcel Service and Federal Express have specific guidelines for shipping such products. It is important to distinguish the category of products, including raw plant, finished herbal product, drug, or a chemical. Each has different regulations, tariff, documentation, and quantity limits.

Identification and Authentication

Plants easily may be confused with other species that are similar in appearance but that are different genetically and chemically. It is difficult to duplicate study results using such plants, and therefore important to know the identity of the study agent. Single botanicals can be identified by their taxonomic nomenclature. The cultivar citation should be included if known.

It is also essential to know the source of raw material captured in the wild, because the properties of a botanical can vary greatly depending on the climate, the geographic region, and the time of harvest.

A qualified botanist then should authenticate the product. The botanical should conform with macroscopic and microscopic descriptions and assays listed in existing literature. The specific parts of the plant used are also important to document, as each part (eg, stem, leaves, flower, roots) contains different bioactive components.

Manufacturing and Processing

Botanical products often are processed to enhance therapeutic effect, to prepare concentrates, and to increase shelf life. Simple extraction with water or alcohol is the most common method used. Manufacturing and processing should follow specific operating procedures that are documented meticulously in the batch records. These specifications include, but are not limited to, weight and the composition of the starting materials, solvent used, processing time and method, excipients used, and the percent yield. If a placebo is used, it should be prepared in the same manner but without the active component.

Quality Control

Unlike synthetic compounds, botanical products may contain active components that vary from batch to batch. It is necessary to have a system according to which agents are standardized. Generally, one or more of the most abundant constituents is selected as a chemical marker for purposes of quality control. Typically, these are compounds that can be detected easily by common laboratory methods such as high pressure liquid chromatography (HPLC) or gas chromatography–mass spectroscopy (GC-MS). For example, hypericin is used as a marker for St. John's wort. Methods such as thin-layer chromatography (TLC) are used commonly for quick fingerprinting, as they are relatively inexpensive and easy to conduct.

Botanical products, however, have many constituents, and the particular constituent selected as the surrogate marker may not contribute to the observed bioactivity. Therefore, it is necessary to develop a bioassay that is relevant to the endpoint for testing the potency of a batch. Such tests must be performed whenever a new lot is used to check for consistency across batches. Tolerance should be predetermined based on previous experience with similar products, and batches that fall outside of the range should be rejected. To avoid potential variation, studies should be planned with a single batch when possible.

The presence of impurities can affect the activity and safety of a product. Impurities may include residues or solvents that cannot be separated during processing, or contaminants such as pesticides, microbials, heavy metals, or adulterants. Every effort must be made to minimize impurities.

Because research may require months or even years, botanical agents may degrade and lose their potency before completion of the study. Proper storage conditions can help prolong shelf life and protect the integrity of the agent. Some products can be kept at room temperature, but others must be stored at lower temperatures and in light-resistant containers in refrigerators. The short- and long-term stability of new agents should be examined; industrial standards on monitoring stability using regular room temperature or accelerated stability studies using higher temperature are available. This information is invaluable to ensure reliable and reproducible data.

The National Center for Complementary and Alternative Medicine (NCCAM) has developed a guidance document to ensure product quality of botanicals and other biologically active agents used in research [25]. The Center for Drug Evaluation and Research (CDER) of FDA provides similar assistance in its "Guidance for Industry for Botanical Drug Products" [26]. There is also an Elaborated CONSORT Statement published recently on reporting randomized, controlled trials of herbal interventions [27]. Not surprisingly, all of these documents contain similar recommendations concerning the identification, manufacture, and quality control of botanical study agents.

The Investigational New Drug Application

A botanical product that shows promising results in preliminary in vitro and animal studies may be investigated further in clinical trials. Because federal law mandates that only approved drugs can be shipped across state lines, the sponsor must get an exemption by submitting an IND application to the FDA. But a botanical study agent can fall in the gray area between a drug and a dietary supplement, in which case an IND may not be required. The FDA, however, recommends IND submission in most cases to ensure monitoring and compliance with proper development and to facilitate any future new drug application process. The FDA also provides a guidance document that is accessible online or through pre-IND meetings with sponsors.

Most botanical products contain multiple ingredients, and in the case of traditional herbal therapies, multiple herbs may be combined into a formula for individual patients. This adds another challenge to IND submission. In theory, each ingredient is considered a separate drug. The FDA, however, does accept a single IND to cover multiple formulations, provided the rationale for such use is justified. Generally, an IND application must provide a description of the product; pharmacology and toxicology data on the agent, or previous experience with the drug in people to demonstrate that the product is reasonably safe for human studies; chemistry and manufacturing information; and a clinical protocol and investigator information.

The CDER has a botanical review team (BRT) to provide resources to address issues related to botanical studies based on "Guidance for Industry Botanical Drug Products" [26,28–33].

CURRENT STATUS AND FUTURE OF BOTANICALS RESEARCH

Funding

Research aimed at new product development typically is supported by industry, and pharmaceutical companies systematically search for new drugs from plant sources. However, most raw botanicals are considered generic products and are not protected by patents. Small companies have little incentive to invest in research to document the efficacy and safety of dietary supplements, as this is not required by law. In addition, negative results could harm sales, and future benefits are not guaranteed. The NCCAM, the US Office of Dietary Supplements (ODS), and other government agencies have supported efforts in academic institutions and other research centers to study dietary supplements including botanicals over the last decade [34]. Research with the greatest potential to impact health, such as that elucidating mechanisms of action, is afforded highest priority.

The NCCAM also emphasizes research that seeks to determine active ingredients, pharmacology, bioavailability and optimal dosing, safety and efficacy, and mechanisms of action.

Current Studies

A survey done on Jan. 29, 2008, revealed 88 botanical clinical trials registered on the NIH Web site [35]. Half of these trials used the randomized, double-blinded, placebo-controlled design that is the accepted gold standard for clinical trials. Interventions in these studies include patented products, mixed herbal formulas, and single herbal extracts, such as green tea (*Camellia sinensis*), black cohosh (*Actaea racemosa* syn. *Cimicifuga racemosa*), St. John's wort, mistletoe (*Viscum album*), and milk thistle (*Silybum marianum*). The safety of herbal products is also an important issue.

SUMMARY

Many herbal supplements are marketed based on their traditional uses. With increasing use of botanicals around the world, information about how they act and their adverse effects, especially when used with modern drugs is needed. Increasing numbers of botanicals are being researched for their safety and efficacy. Botanicals research, however, has its unique issues, ranging from product standardization to study design. Obtaining funding for research is also a challenge, but over the last decade, governmental agencies have begun supporting high-quality botanicals research. As a result of such efforts, the number of studies involving botanicals has increased. There is also a rise in the number of clinical trials of herbs for cancer treatment, prevention, and improvement of quality of life in cancer patients. This trend is encouraging, and future studies likely will unravel the mechanisms of action leading to development of new drugs and increase acceptance of botanical dietary supplements in cancer therapies. Evidence-based research also will help ensure the safety and efficacy of botanical dietary supplements.

References

[1] Kelly JP, Kaufman DW, Kelley K, et al. Use of herbal/natural supplements according to racial/ethnic group. J Altern Complement Med 2006;12(6):555–61.

[2] Correa-Velez I, Clavarino A, Eastwood H. Surviving, relieving, repairing, and boosting up: reasons for using complementary/alternative medicine among patients with advanced cancer: a thematic analysis. J Palliat Med 2005;8(5):953–61.

[3] Gupta D, Lis CG, Birdsall TC, et al. The use of dietary supplements in a community hospital comprehensive cancer center: implications for conventional cancer care. Support Care Cancer 2005;13(11):912–9.

[4] Evans M, Shaw A, Thompson EA, et al. Decisions to use complementary and alternative medicine (CAM) by male cancer patients: information-seeking roles and types of evidence used. BMC Complement Altern Med 2007;7:25.

[5] Verhoef MJ, Balneaves LG, Boon HS, et al. Reasons for and characteristics associated with complementary and alternative medicine use among adult cancer patients: a systematic review. Integr Cancer Ther 2005;4(4):274–86.

[6] Meijerman I, Beijnen JH, Schellens JH. Herb–drug interactions in oncology: focus on mechanisms of induction. Oncologist 2006;11(7):742–52.

[7] Yeung KS, Gubili J. Clinical guide to herb–drug interactions in oncology. J Soc Integr Oncol 2007;5(3):113–7.

[8] Linde K, Mulrow CD, Berner M, et al. St John's wort for depression. Cochrane Database Syst Rev 2005;(2):CD000448.

[9] Mathijssen RH, Verweij J, de Bruijn P, et al. Effects of St. John's wort on irinotecan metabolism. J Natl Cancer Inst 2002;94(16):1247–9.

[10] Chinese Pharmacopoeia Commission. Pharmacopoeia of the People's Republic of China. Beijing (China): People's Medical Publishing House; 2005.

[11] Blumenthal M, editor. The Complete German Commission E Monographs—Therapeutic Guide to Herbal Medicines. Boston: Integrative Medicine Communications; 1998.

[12] Ekins S, Mestres J, Testa B. In silico pharmacology for drug discovery: applications to targets and beyond. Br J Pharmacol 2007;152(1):21–37.

[13] NCI/NIH. Developmental therapeutics program. Available at: http://dtp.nci.nih.gov/branches/npb/repository.html. Accessed January 29, 2008.

[14] NCI/NIH. Natural products branch. Available at: http://dtp.nci.nih.gov/screening.html. Accessed January 29, 2008.

[15] Cragg GM, Boyd MR, Cardellina JH 2nd, et al. Ethnobotany and drug discovery: the experience of the US National Cancer Institute. Ciba Found Symp 1994;185:178–90 [discussion: 190–76].

[16] WHO. General guidelines for methodologies on research and evaluation of traditional medicine. Available at: http://whqlibdoc.who.int/hq/2000/WHO_EDM_TRM_2000.1.pdf. Accessed January 29, 2008.

[17] Hishida I, Nanba H, Kuroda H. Antitumor activity exhibited by orally administered extract from fruit body of Grifola frondosa (maitake). Chem Pharm Bull (Tokyo) 1988;36(5):1819–27.

[18] Vickers AJ. How to design a phase I trial of an anticancer botanical. J Soc Integr Oncol 2006;4(1):46–51.

[19] Daugherty CK, Ratain MJ, Emanuel EJ, et al. Ethical, scientific, and regulatory perspectives regarding the use of placebos in cancer clinical trials. J Clin Oncol 2008;26(8):1371–8.

[20] Newton KM, Reed SD, LaCroix AZ, et al. Treatment of vasomotor symptoms of menopause with black cohosh, multibotanicals, soy, hormone therapy, or placebo: a randomized trial. Ann Intern Med 2006;145(12):869–79.

[21] Pockaj BA, Gallagher JG, Loprinzi CL, et al. Phase III double-blind, randomized, placebo-controlled crossover trial of black cohosh in the management of hot flashes: NCCTG Trial N01CC1. J Clin Oncol 2006;24(18):2836–41.

[22] USDA. Fresh product grading and quality certification. Available at: http://www.ams.usda.gov/fv/fpbgapghp.htm. Accessed January 29, 2008.

[23] WHO. WHO guidelines on good agricultural and collection practices (GACP) for medicinal plants. Available at: http://whqlibdoc.who.int/publications/2003/9241546271.pdf. Accessed January 29, 2008.

[24] FDA. Current good manufacturing practice in manufacturing, packaging, labeling, or holding operations for dietary supplements. Available at: http://www.fda.gov/OHRMS/DOCKETS/98fr/07-3039.pdf. Accessed February 27, 2008.

[25] NCCAM. Interim applicant guidance: product quality: biologically active agents used in complementary and alternative medicine (CAM) and placebo materials. Available at: http://grants.nih.gov/grants/guide/notice-files/NOT-AT-05-004.html. Accessed January 29, 2008.

[26] CDER. Guidance for industry–botanical drug products. Available at: http://www.fda.gov/cder/index.html. Accessed January 29, 2008.

[27] Gagnier JJ, Boon H, Rochon P, et al. Reporting randomized, controlled trials of herbal interventions: an elaborated CONSORT statement. Ann Intern Med 2006;144(5):364–7.

[28] CDER. Guidance for industry: formal meetings with sponsors and applicants for PDUFA products. Available at: http://www.fda.gov/cder/guidance/2125fnl.pdf. Accessed January 29, 2008.

[29] CDER. Botanical review team. Available at: http://www.fda.gov/cder/index.html. Accessed January 29, 2008.

[30] CDER. Guidance documents. Available at: www.fda.gov/cder/guidance/index.htm. Accessed January 29, 2008.

[31] CDER. Guidance for industry–botanical drug products. Available at: http://www.fda.gov/cder/guidance/4592fnl.pdf. Accessed January 29, 2008.

[32] CDER. Drug applications. Available at: http://www.fda.gov/cder/regulatory/applications/ind_page_1.htm. Accessed January 29, 2008.

[33] CDER. Drug approval application process. Available at: http://www.fda.gov/cder/regulatory/applications/default.htm. Accessed January 29, 2008.

[34] NCCAM. NCCAM's research centers program. Available at: http://nccam.nih.gov/training/centers/. Accessed January 31, 2008.

[35] NIH. Clinical trials. Available at: http://www.clinicaltrials.gov/. Accessed January 29, 2008.

Hematol Oncol Clin N Am 22 (2008) 671–682

HEMATOLOGY/ONCOLOGY CLINICS
OF NORTH AMERICA

From Studying Patient Treatment to Studying Patient Care: Arriving at Methodologic Crossroads

Marja J. Verhoef, PhD[a],*, Anne Leis, PhD[b]

[a]Department of Community Health Sciences, University of Calgary, 3330 Hospital Drive NW, Calgary, Alberta, Canada, T2N 4N1
[b]Department of Community Health and Epidemiology, 107 Wiggins Road, University of Saskatchewan, Saskatoon, Saskatchewan, Canada, S7N 5E5

Many factors have contributed to the increasing recognition of the importance of cancer care that moves beyond a primary focus on cancer diagnosis and treatment. These factors include the evolving chronic nature of cancer, the increase in survivorship and the related research and treatment emphasis, the recognition that outcomes other than survival are important and valuable, and patients' increased desire for participation in cancer management. Cancer care is more than treatment and refers to the multiple interacting ways to support a patient and his or her family during the assessment, treatment, and follow-up of his or her disease in addition to the assessment of and response to associated consequences. Cancer care also includes support for patients' decision to use complementary and alternative medicine (CAM) therapies or products or to engage in lifestyle behaviors, such as changing diet or exercise behavior. The increased use of CAM by patients who have cancer in addition to conventional treatment has highlighted the importance that patients attach to a comprehensive multidisciplinary approach to cancer care and to outcomes other than survival, suggesting that some patients seek healing in addition to, or instead of, curing. Healing is a dynamic process of recovery, repair, restoration, reintegration, renewal, and transformation that increases resilience, coherence, and wholeness. It is an emergent process of the person's whole system (physical, mental, social, spiritual, and environmental) and a unique personal and communal process that may or may not involve curing [1].

Barabási [2] suggests that most twentieth century research has been driven by reductionism: the process of attempting to understand a problem by first deciphering its components. Cancer research seems to be no exception. To date, cancer research has mostly but not exclusively focused on assessing and evaluating biomedical cancer treatments through reductionist methodologies, such as

*Corresponding author. E-mail address: mverhoef@ucalgary.ca (M.J. Verhoef).

0889-8588/08/$ – see front matter
doi:10.1016/j.hoc.2008.04.006
hemonc.theclinics.com

randomized controlled trials (RCTs). Yet, given the complex nature of cancer care, a new research perspective is needed to address its multilayered character.

The objectives of this article are (1) to discuss the evolving nature of cancer care, (2) to address the challenges faced by biomedical research methodology when applied to cancer care, and (3) to identify new research directions to meet these challenges.

CANCER CARE

Cancer care is multifactorial and patient centered. It can be described as a complex package or "bundle" [3] of interventions, delivered at different times and places with different intentions, that interacts and cannot be evaluated in isolation. It interacts with the patient's unique context and is a process potentially resulting in a wide range of outcomes. Depending on the individual and his or her context, it may include medical treatments (eg, radiation, chemotherapy, surgery), psychosocial interventions (eg, mind-body therapies, support groups), complementary therapies (eg, natural health products, massage therapy, acupuncture), alternative systems of care (eg, traditional Chinese medicine, naturopathic medicine), and self-care (eg, lifestyle behaviors). Some interventions are offered by health care professionals at an oncology center, and others are provided by complementary practitioners or are selected by patients without consulting practitioners. This means that cancer care is situated at the crossroads of diverse professional systems, lay referral and support networks, and the "self-care" industry. The patient is at the center of several care and support systems that are embedded in the larger social, cultural, political, and economic systems of which the patient is a part. In such a view, multiple interactions among the various systems have a cumulative and synergistic impact on the patient's healing journey. This interplay between the patient and these various systems defines the dynamic nature of cancer care. Cancer care with the patient at its core is a dynamic, adaptive, nonlinear process responding to the patient's changing needs over time. Cancer care differs for each patient, because of the unique context in which care takes place, which includes the patient's values, beliefs, expectations, physical condition, personality, and meaning he or she gives to treatment. Further, for each patient, cancer care differs at diagnosis, during treatment, during follow-up, and as he or she becomes a survivor.

A promising move toward a focus on cancer care rather than on biomedical treatments comes from the relatively new discipline of integrative oncology, which seems to reflect a shift in focus from biomedical cancer treatment to the more comprehensive concept of cancer care. The authors of *Integrative Oncology Practice Guidelines* [4] define this approach as "the ability to integrate the best of complementary and mainstream care using a multidisciplinary approach, combining the best of mainstream cancer care and rational, data-based, adjunctive complementary therapies." Sagar [5], in line with what the authors outlined previously, argues that the aim of integrative oncology should be one medicine that synergistically combines therapies and services in "a manner that exceeds the collaborative effort of the individual practices." When considering the philosophy of integrative oncology, Mumber [6] views integrative oncology as an approach to cancer care that addresses all participants at all levels of their being and experience. It is the next step in the evolution of cancer care that "espouses a renewed focus on the guiding principles of medicine, emphasizing healing over curing."

Despite this shift toward integrative cancer care, research programs have yet to address the challenges that this emerging discipline introduces for the investigation of cancer care, specifically the need for new methodologic approaches. Cancer care and integrative oncology are inherently complex and challenge established research methodologies to be able to answer the most important research questions. A new research framework is needed to address the complexities of cancer care, to do justice to the comprehensiveness of the approach, and, ultimately, to improve cancer management and the well-being of patients.

METHODOLOGIC CHALLENGES

In the literature, integrative oncology is often described as an evidence-based discipline [4–7], but researchers often draw on reductionist notions of evidence that may be appropriate to assess cancer treatments but contradict the notion of integrative oncology. The difficult questions of what evidence is and how it can be established for this emerging discipline remain, for a major part, unasked and therefore unanswered.

The value of scientific evidence for informing clinical treatment decisions derives for the most part from experimental design features, as applied in RCTs (eg, control groups, randomization, blinding, standardized patient selection criteria, standardized treatments). The RCT is designed for relatively straightforward standardized interventions, however, and is applicable only under highly controlled circumstances. It is questionable how relevant and applicable an RCT is to highly individualized complex interventions, such as integrative oncology and cancer care in natural environments [8,9]. This viewpoint indeed faces major challenges, some of which are listed in Table 1. Primarily scientific evidence derived from RCTs provides a narrow view of what constitutes "good" evidence. RCTs typically exclude potentially important and informative qualitative and observational data about the use and benefits of an intervention in real-world settings. Along with his colleagues, Sackett (one of the leaders in promoting evidence-based medicine [EBM]), initially defined evidence as the integration of individual clinical expertise with the best external evidence from systematic research [11]. However, a few years later, they reframed this definition as "the integration of the best research evidence with clinical expertise and patient values" [12]. This definition highlights that clinical expertise based, in part, on empiric observation may provide important information beyond what can be learned from clinical trials. In addition, it highlights that the patient has important knowledge that is unavailable to the health care provider. Although clinical expertise and patient values are limited by their subjective nature, scientific evidence is limited by its objectivity and attempt to control but not to account for important subjective factors.

Table 1
Challenges to randomized controlled trial designs when evaluating complex interventions

Standardization	It is extremely difficult to standardize multifactorial individualized cancer care. Attempting to do so may result in a trial that does not accurately reflect the nature of the intervention.
Randomization	Patients choosing an integrated care approach often make a well-considered decision built on strong treatment preferences and high expectations. Therefore, only a limited group of patients may agree to randomization, which may have an impact on the validity of trial results.
Blinding	Blinding and finding appropriate placebos are impossible for cancer care, which consists of multiple, individualized, interacting components.
Results apply to groups only	RCTs provide an estimate of the average patient response only and give little or no information on how a specific patient reacts to a specific treatment. This means that exceptional patients "disappear" in the trial and important determinants of "doing well" (or not) cannot be identified.
Placebo effects	RCTs are designed to avoid nonspecific and placebo effects, which may include effects of the patient-provider relationship, attention, compassion, modulation of anxiety, and patient and practitioner expectations. These elements are considered fundamental to many CAM and integrative care approaches because they have the potential to enhance the intervention and to increase the therapeutic response [10] but cannot be measured through an RCT design.

In combination, scientific evidence, clinical expertise, and patient values greatly contribute to optimal evidence-based patient care.

This perspective does not discount the benefits of the RCT design. In many but not all circumstances, scientific evidence may best be acquired through the use of the RCT design; however, assessment of clinical expertise and patient values requires a different approach. The need for a variety of types of evidence is also supported by the Canadian Health Services Research Foundation (CHSRF), although in different terms. The CHSRF has published an insightful report [13] that distinguishes between context-free scientific evidence; context-sensitive evidence; and the expertise, views, and realities of stakeholders. Context-sensitive evidence is derived from the social sciences on the premise that evidence has little meaning or importance for decision making if it is not adapted to the circumstances of its application. Context-sensitive evidence is what is required to assess cancer care appropriately in a manner that privileges all stakeholders' perspectives.

A further consideration in the drive to develop evidence related to cancer care is how patients use that evidence. Interviews with patients who have cancer have demonstrated that, given their own context, they seek a wide and different range of sources of evidence, of which scientific evidence is only a part [14]. New users of CAM tended to do so to address side effects and to improve their quality of life. They valued scientific evidence and were concerned about safety. They looked for credible sources and consistency of information among sources. Alternatively, those who had a history of CAM use considered this as part of their wellness regimen and believed strongly in CAM's positive effects. They were more likely to follow personal experience and their gut feelings rather than scientific evidence. Furthermore, patients who had late-stage cancer saw CAM as a strategy to maintain hope, to gain control, and to extend life. They were willing to try anything that sounded promising. For this group, risks associated with CAM treatments were usually not an important factor. They valued magazines, television programs, and testimonials as evidence sources.

What this review tells us is that evidence itself is a subjective concept, with different definitions for different stakeholders depending on their purpose. It also highlights that multiple perspectives are needed when assessing cancer care. The need for holistic evidence that acknowledges the complex, multifactorial, individualized, dynamic, and nonlinear nature of cancer care begs the question of how cancer care can be evaluated.

METHODOLOGIC DIRECTIONS TO EVALUATING CANCER CARE

In this section, the authors first focus on qualitative research, particularly the need to combine qualitative research with quantitative methods, including RCTs. They then discuss a more recent methodologic approach labeled whole systems research and end with potential research directions.

Qualitative Research

Qualitative research is the investigation of phenomena in their natural context, typically in an in-depth and holistic fashion, through the collection of rich narrative materials using a flexible research design. Its purpose is exploration and acquisition of in-depth understanding of participants' motives, thoughts, and behaviors [15]. Qualitative research is eminently suitable to help improve our understanding of the systems and related interactions within cancer care. For example, there is a need to understand how a package of cancer care is developed from among the many potential therapeutic and self-care approaches, how that package changes over time, and why many patients who have cancer have such strong beliefs in comprehensive and integrated cancer treatment and care. Such research allows the development of testable explanations (hypotheses) about how, when, and why cancer care or its elements work. Despite its nonnumeric data, qualitative analysis is rigorous and follows strict rules [16]. The authors present some examples of results from their qualitative studies as a means to illustrate how qualitative research has contributed to their understanding of cancer care and what is taking place at the individual patient level. Quotes from study participants illustrating these results are included in Table 2.

1. Individual outcomes: Patients often describe the outcomes of integrative cancer treatment and care in terms of outcomes that move beyond the often used biomedical and quality-of-life measures. In addition to these more common outcomes, the authors' results demonstrate the importance of physical,

psychologic, social, spiritual, and holistic outcomes and highlight that out-comes most important to a given patient are individualized to that person's perspective and goals [17,18].

2. Links between process and outcome of care: The results of the authors' inter-views demonstrate that the process and context of cancer care are intercon-nected and have an impact on patient outcomes.

3. Meaning shifts: The process of care often involves a shift in the meaning that a patient gives to the intervention. Stibich and Wissow [19] have described that acupuncture students identified five different types of meaning shifts after wellness acupuncture over time: (1) from the goal of fixing the problem to the goal of increasing health, (2) from symptoms as problems to symptoms as teachers, (3) from healing as passive to healing as active, (4) from being dominated by illness to moving beyond illness, and (5) from regarding the practitioner as a technician to regarding the practitioner as a healer. When the authors conducted a secondary analysis of transcripts of inter-views with patients receiving integrative cancer care, they found each shift to be identified by patients who had cancer as well.

Being aware of these shifts allows practitioners to interact with patients at their level of understanding and interpretation. In addition, it allows reframing the can-cer experience and being able to find healing even when the primary condition is untreatable. Thus, meaning shifts may have important therapeutic value.

The Value-Added of a Combined Methods Approach

Given the insights that qualitative research provides about cancer care and healing experiences, it would be beneficial to add such data collection to quan-titative studies. One example is to complement RCTs with qualitative methods to identify how patients benefit in addition to assessing quantitatively whether improvement occurs. Only a few such studies have been conducted in the cancer field. In one study [20], an RCT was conducted to identify whether hyp-notherapy reduces anxiety and improves quality of life in patients who have cancer and are undergoing curative radiotherapy. In addition, study partici-pants were interviewed and completed a questionnaire to ascertain their opin-ions about the therapy. The investigators identified, among other results, that the Short Form-36 (SF-36) might have been too insensitive to detect changes in well-being. Individual interviews clarified that the observed improvement in sense of well-being may not have been derived from the hypnotherapy but instead from the patient-practitioner relationship and from seeing cancer as a challenge to make the best of life. This example indicates how elements of care other than the intervention can have an impact on patient outcomes and can identify changes that would have been missed without the qualitative component.

Similarly, adding qualitative interviews or focus groups to observational stud-ies contributes to understanding dynamic cancer care decisions better over time and may lead to useful information for clinicians. In the authors' mixed methods study of women who have breast cancer (ongoing) and declined at least one of the conventional treatments they have been offered, they added focus groups

Table 2
Illustrations of qualitative study results

Theme	Illustrative quote
Wide range of nonconventional outcomes	"I am changed, and so the way I do things in my life is different. My whole pace has slowed down, so how I organize my day is different... I am more present in my life. Overall, I guess I just really, I feel different. I even think I look different. This has been a very profound and wonderful experience for me."
Links between context, process, and outcomes	"The [integrative clinic] has built a healing community like no other. The dedication, positive loving attitude and hard work have created an oasis of peace, a place where healing can blossom, a place where people with illnesses have become partners in their own health process, a place of wholeness. You have given us hope, where others only gave us numbers. You have given us back our lives."
Meaning shift (from healing as passive to healing as active)	"I am watching but not waiting. I really am pointedly looking for the best things I can do everyday from 5 minutes of doing a tiny bit of relaxation, visualization on the thoughts about how the white blood cells are gobbling up my cancer... I am doing all those kinds of things and many more. Next week I am going on a retreat for people who have had exactly this kind of cancer and a major life decision. I am doing everything I possibly can. I am using up some of my holidays to do that. I have changed my job. Changed aspects of my job, not changed my job completely to improve my lifestyle to try and turn this thing around with my body and work with my body as it works against it."
Meaning shift (from being dominated by illness to moving beyond illness)	"Sure, this isn't the way I imagined things turning out for me but the major turning point for me was, I think, realizing that and accepting that. We had a ritual in the group that we did to kind of make amends with our bodies and cancer. It was what was so life altering. I still feel scared at times, sure, but I would say now that I feel more confident and a lot more calm."

These interviews are based on the authors' interviews conducted with patients who have cancer and were attending integrative health care centers in Canada.

and personal interviews to a longitudinal case-controlled quantitative study. The purposes were (1) to validate the authors' analysis of the interview data, and (2) to have the women develop what they thought were the most important recommendations for health professionals. The two most important recommendations were to reduce stress at early diagnosis and to facilitate access to truly integrative cancer care. Many concrete suggestions were provided. Such data help in further enhancing cancer care.

Whole Systems Research

Beyond adding qualitative research to quantitative studies, there is even more to gain by approaching research design through a systems perspective. A whole system can be described as an approach to health care in which practitioners apply bodies of knowledge and associated practices to maximize the patient's capacity to achieve mental and physical balance and restore his or her own health, using individualized nonreductionist approaches to diagnosis and treatment [21]. Examples are traditional Chinese medicine, in addition to more conventional approaches, such as addiction treatment and palliative care. Rather than a research design, whole systems research is better described as an "emerging research framework specifically designed for the evaluation of complex multimodal interventions" [22]. This means that all elements of an intervention, including its context (eg, setting, provider characteristics) and process (eg, patient-provider communication) are part of the "whole" intervention. In regard to a whole system, nothing is irrelevant. Therefore, whole systems research aims at appropriately combining and integrating qualitative and quantitative research designs and methods in a coherent research program so that all aspects of an internally consistent approach to treatment, or a whole system, can be assessed.

When researchers first raised the notion of whole system interventions within CAM [21], they were primarily thinking about established CAM systems, such as traditional Chinese medicine, naturopathy, or homeopathy. Over the past few years, however, the notion of whole systems has been extended to other systems, for example, integrative medicine that combines treatments from conventional medicine and CAM in a unique system of practitioners and modalities. Similarly, in choosing CAM treatments to supplement conventional cancer treatment, individuals also seem to be establishing their own system [23]. Accordingly, cancer care is not one single system that has a specific beginning and an end but consists of multiple interacting systems that affect each other. Cancer care finds itself embedded and entangled in additional layers of complexity at the individual, oncology care system, and policy levels that could be described within an ecologic framework. As such, cancer care meets the characteristics of what Holden [24] describes as a complex adaptive system with the complexity of the therapeutic encounter and the therapies themselves.

When studying cancer care, several whole systems research principles are helpful to consider (Table 3). Investigators must remain flexible and adaptive through this process, moving iteratively among phases as appropriate and as

Table 3
Whole systems research as a process

Phase 1	Recognition of underlying assumptions of cancer care, for example, holism and patient centeredness
Phase 2	Careful exploration and description of all aspects of cancer care and desired outcomes at patient, practitioner, and policy levels
Phase 3	Description of the process and context of cancer care in unique environments
Phase 4	Identification of patterns of treatment and care between patients and settings
Phase 5	Development of testable explanations of observed processes, contexts, and outcomes (conceptual models)
Phase 6	Testing these explanations

new knowledge is gained. Often, this process is nonsequential and can generate untapped information that has the potential to enhance cancer care.

For the first phases of this process, Aickin [25] and Fønnebø [26] have provided useful suggestions. Early phase research consists of studies using a small number of participants and a large number of variables to document the processes and context of cancer care better and to identify patterns. Results of such studies allow formulation and testing of hypotheses through more or less traditional means. The aim of early phase research can be seen as refining the (ultimate) design by making errors. More specifically it looks at the appropriateness of the study group, willingness to be recruited, appropriateness and reliability of outcomes, treatments used, assessment of nonspecific effects, and the impact of those who deliver care. Most likely, the amount of information obtained from early phase research is so substantial that a single subsequent hypothesis testing study would not be sufficient; instead, a program of research consisting of several studies is likely to emerge.

To factor in the whole system's indivisible, adaptive, dynamic characteristics in addition to the nonlinear interactions among components, the next phases of the whole systems research process must turn to innovative approaches to evaluate individualized care within its unique context. Currently, not much is known about the nature of specific whole system interventions; however, a systems thinking approach may contain some of the key elements likely to influence and inform the next steps of the research. Systems thinking represents a way of viewing how systems behave from a broad perspective that includes examining overall structures, patterns, and cycles rather than considering only specific and separate systems or components of systems. A wide array of methods and tools grounded in the combination of quantitative, qualitative, and participatory methodologies (eg, computer simulation modeling; quantitative, qualitative, and metaphoric approaches; concept mapping) can be used to complement linear thinking and reductionist methods of inquiry [27]. The following two examples illustrate what these next steps might look like.

A case study in which the case is a specific issue or problem arising in the cancer care system may be a promising approach to capture some critical aspects of this system [28]. A case study can not only document and analyze people's knowledge, attitudes, actions, and beliefs within each system of cancer care but also looks for system characteristics, such as the nature and patterns of interactions, to understand the problem at stake better and find an appropriate course of action. An example is the issue of missed cancer care appointments in a particular setting. A complex systems view searches beyond assessing patient-related factors and also looks at systemic factors (eg, processes, tensions, contradictions). Instead of solely blaming a part of the system, such as patients, a novel and perhaps unexpected approach to the issue becomes possible.

Participatory methods, such as needs assessments, brainstorming, open space meeting, concept mapping, and participatory community development, can also be used to examine complex problems occurring in the cancer care system. In contrast to case study methodology, this approach is not only researcher driven but engages all people working, behaving, interacting, and adapting within a component or system of the cancer care system (ie, patients, health care providers, front-line workers, decision makers) as partners and experts in the research process [29]. Key stakeholders' engagement and their expertise combined with their insights drive the systems' study and the analysis and facilitate the emergence of a renewed vision for cancer care or the description of novel models of care. Thus, with its broad application from biology [30] to the social environment [31], the systems thinking perspective seems to offer promising and unprecedented insights into the complex adaptive system of cancer care and may create exciting directions for system change.

SUMMARY

As the authors argue throughout this article, cancer care is best viewed as a system of interacting components that includes diverse professional systems, lay referral and support networks, and the "self-care" industry, with the patient and all his or her characteristics at the center. This perspective is beginning to be acknowledged in the oncology system, most notably through the emerging discipline of integrative oncology. Integrative oncology practice recognizes that cancer care is more than treatment and includes life management and the means to integrate fragmented care. Ideally, what is desired is an answer to the question of what type of cancer care works and works better than others.

There is a need to consider alternative approaches to studying cancer care and to acknowledge that cancer care is much more than a specific intervention. Such approaches are only beginning to be developed. Although many investigators recognize the shortcomings of RCTs for the evaluation of complex interventions, they have difficulty in identifying new approaches [7]. This means that we have arrived at the crossroads, because the new approaches that the authors suggest are extremely useful in understanding complex interventions and cancer care; however, they do not result in being able to identify a causal relation between care and common medical and quality-of-life outcomes. In other words, such approaches do not result in scientific evidence but are instrumental in providing context-related evidence.

Although oncology researchers may thus consider such research as irrelevant, it is important to recognize and document how patients approach their cancer management. Attention to the importance of lifestyle behaviors is increasing, and many patients add CAM to their treatment regimen. The range of these CAM treatments is extremely wide and varies from systems, such as homeopathy, to professions, such as manipulative and body-based medicine and energy medicine, to herbal treatments, to mind-body interventions. Ideally, these components of cancer care should not be looked at in isolation but be coordinated as a comprehensive, balanced, and individualized treatment package. Such packages should be evaluated in a comprehensive manner.

Because the authors' focus was on research designs to assess whether cancer care benefits patients, issues of safety and risk have not been addressed. The authors recognize that these cannot be ignored and are extremely important, because combining different types of treatment may involve risk. This topic, however, was not the purpose of this article.

An interdisciplinary program of research would be a helpful start to begin to discuss the type of evidence needed and the appropriate research approaches to obtain such evidence. Such a program should be based on collaboration and the desire to benefit from combined expertise to avoid duplication. Differences of opinion should be cherished because they may lead to diverse views to study similar issues, which may result in an improved understanding of the benefits of each approach.

This article has focused mostly on the patients' perspective and has touched on the researchers' perspective. It is also essential to include a wide range of medical, CAM, and allied health professionals in such discussions.

Acknowledgment

The authors thank Laura Weeks, PhD (candidate), for her careful review of the manuscript and her helpful suggestions.

References

[1] Jonas WB, Chez RA, Duffy B, et al. Investigating the impact of optimal healing environments. Altern Ther Health Med 2003;9(6):36–40.

[2] Barabási AL. Linked: the new science of networks. New York: Perseus Books; 2002.

[3] Institute of Medicine of the National Academies. Need for innovative designs in research on CAM and conventional medicine. Complementary and alternative medicine in the United States. Washington, DC: National Academies Press; 2005. p. 108–128.

[4] Deng GE, Cassileth BR, Cohen L, et al. Integrative oncology practice guidelines. J Soc Integr Oncol 2007;5(2):65–84.

[5] Sagar SM. Integrative oncology in North America. J Soc Integr Oncol 2006;4(1):27–39.

[6] Mumber M. Integrative oncology: an overview. In: Rakel D, editor. Integrative medicine. Philadelphia: Saunders Elsevier; 2007. p. 811–20.

[7] Berk LB. Primer on integrative oncology. Hematol Oncol Clin North Am 2006;20(1): 213–31.

[8] Walach H, Jonas WB, Lewith G. The role of outcomes research in evaluating complementary and alternative medicine. In: Lewith G, Jonas WB, Walach H, editors. Clinical research in complementary therapies: principles, problems and solutions. Edinburgh (Midlothian): Churchill Livingstone; 2002. p. 29–45.

[9] Moerman DE, Jonas WB. Deconstructing the placebo effect and finding the meaning response. Ann Intern Med 2002;136(6):471–6.

[10] Block KI, Burns B, Cohen AJ, et al. Point-counterpoint: using clinical trials for the evaluation of integrative cancer therapies. Integr Cancer Ther 2004;3(1):66–81.

[11] Sackett DL, Rosenberg W, Gray J, et al. Evidence based medicine: what it is and what it isn't. BMJ 1996;312:71–2.

[12] Sackett DL, Straus SE, Richardson WS, et al. Evidence-based medicine: how to practice and teach EBM. 2nd edition. London: Churchill Livingstone; 2000.

[13] Limas J, Culyer T, McCutcheon C, et al. Conceptualizing and combining evidence for health system guidance. Ottawa (ON): Canadian Health Services Research Foundation; 2005. p. 1–44.

[14] Verhoef MJ, Mulkins A, Carlson LE, et al. Assessing the role of evidence in patients' evaluation of complementary therapies: a quality study. Integr Cancer Ther 2007;6(4):345–53.

[15] Polit DF, Hungler BP. Nursing research: principles and methods. 6th edition. Philadelphia: Lippincott; 1999.

[16] Krefting L. Rigor in qualitative research: the assessment of trustworthiness. Am J Occup Ther 1990;45(3):214–22.

[17] Verhoef MJ, Mulkins A, Boon H. Integrative health care: how can we determine whether patients benefit? J Altern Complement Med 2005;11(Suppl 1):S57–65.

[18] Verhoef MJ, Vanderheyden L, Dryden T, et al. Evaluating complementary and alternative medicine interventions: in search of appropriate patient-centred outcome measures. BMC Complement Altern Med 2006;6:3810.1186/1472-2882-6-38.

[19] Stibich M, Wissow L. Meaning shift: findings from wellness acupuncture. Altern Ther Health Med 2006;12(2):42–8.

[20] Stalpers LJ, da Costa HC, Merbis MA, et al. Hypnotherapy in radiotherapy patients: a randomized trial. Int J Radiat Oncol Biol Phys 2005;61(2):499–506.

[21] Ritenbaugh C, Verhoef M, Fleishman S, et al. Whole systems research: a discipline for studying complementary and alternative medicine. Altern Ther Health Med 2003;9(4):32–6.

[22] Verhoef MJ, Lewith G, Ritenbaugh C, et al. Complementary and alternative medicine whole systems research: beyond identification of inadequacies of the RCT. Complement Ther Med 2005;13(3):206–12.

[23] Ritenbaugh C. Guiding concepts for whole systems research. In: Whole systems research in cancer care—report of a meeting in Tromsø (Sommarøy). Complement Ther Med 2006;14:161–64.

[24] Holden LM. Complex adaptive systems: concept analysis. J Adv Nurs 2005;52(6):651–7.

[25] Aickin M. The importance of early phase research. J Altern Complement Med 2007;13(4):447–50.

[26] Fønnebø V. Early phase research is needed in CAM and conventional medicine endeavors. J Altern Complement Med 2007;13(4):397–8.

[27] von Bertalanffy L. General system theory: foundations, development, applications. New York: George Braziller; 1968. p. pxxii.

[28] Anderson RA, Crabtree BF, Steele DJ, et al. Case study: the view from complexity science. Qual Health Res 2005;15(5):669–85.

[29] Trochim WM, Milstein B, Wood BJ, et al. Setting objectives for community and systems change: an application of concept mapping for planning a statewide health improvement initiative. Health Promot Pract 2004;5(1):8–19.

[30] Janecka IP. Cancer control through principles of systems science, complexity and chaos theory: a model. Int J Med Sci 2007;4(3):164–73.

[31] Gatrell AC. Complexity theory and geographies of health: a critical assessment. Soc Sci Med 2005;60:2661–71.

Hematol Oncol Clin N Am 22 (2008) 683–708

HEMATOLOGY/ONCOLOGY CLINICS
OF NORTH AMERICA

Mind-Body Medicine and Cancer

James S. Gordon, MD[a,b,c,d,*]

[a]The Center for Mind-Body Medicine, 5225 Connecticut Avenue NW, Suite 414,
Washington, DC 20015, USA
[b]Department of Psychiatry, Georgetown University School of Medicine, Georgetown University
Medical Center, 4000 Reservoir Road NW, Suite 120, Washington, DC 20007, USA
[c]Department of Family Medicine, Georgetown University School of Medicine, Georgetown
University Medical Center, 4000 Reservoir Road NW, Suite 120, Washington, DC 20007, USA
[d]CancerGuides® Training Program, 5225 Connecticut Avenue NW, Suite 414,
Washington, DC 20015, USA

Ten years ago, two of my students at Georgetown Medical School volunteered to do a presentation on "mind-body medicine and cancer." It was the last session of a semester-long elective on integrative medicine and one they felt highly qualified to lead. Both were budding scientists and had done summer laboratory research at the National Cancer Institute, and both were, they told us, highly skeptical of the mind-body connection. Therapeutic answers to cancer, they believed, lay in genetics and molecular biology, and in the next generation of precisely targeted chemotherapeutic agents. They would, they promised us, cast a cool, critical eye on these mind-body alternatives that seemed at first glance to be such unlikely therapeutic interventions. I assigned the topic to them and waited with interest to hear what they would say.

As their fellow first-year students made their weekly presentations—on the relationship between stress and chronic illness, nutrition and heart disease, and the principles and practices of Chinese medicine—the two young scientists listened carefully and asked hard, thoughtful questions.

On the last afternoon of class, it was their turn. When the class assembled, they had already covered the board with diagrams of the interactions between the mind, brain, and immune system, and with citations from journal articles. They took us swiftly and skillfully through the physiology and biochemistry and then turned their attention to the clinical research. They handed out sheets of references: Relaxation techniques and guided imagery, they showed us, improved the quality of life for people who had cancer, decreased the nausea and vomiting of chemotherapy and the pain of metastatic disease, and enhanced the numbers and functioning of immune cells. "Much to our surprise," one of them concluded, "the connections are clear and the hard science is there.

*The Center for Mind-Body Medicine, 5225 Connecticut Avenue NW, Suite 414, Washington,
DC 20015. E-mail address: jgordon@cmbm.org

0889-8588/08/$ – see front matter
doi:10.1016/j.hoc.2008.04.010

The evidence tells us that mind-body medicine should be as central to cancer care as chemotherapy and radiation. Every oncologist should know about it. And every patient should have mind-body approaches available as soon as he has been diagnosed."

The research that has been done in the last 10 years, the papers that have been published, and the experience of hundreds, perhaps thousands, of clinicians and hundreds of thousands of patients now confirm and amplify my skeptical students' hard-won conclusions. Mind-body medicine, grounded in a respectful, therapeutic partnership, facilitating each patient's involvement in his or her own treatment, and emphasizing the capacity to positively affect his or her illness, should be a central element in the care of every person diagnosed with cancer.

This article reviews some of the physiologic foundations of mind-body medicine, the introduction of mind-body approaches to cancer care in the 1970s, the specific mind-body approaches that have been used, and the evidence that supports their use. The importance of group support for enhancing the effectiveness of these approaches is discussed, and the article concludes by offering some guidelines for integrating mind-body approaches and perspectives in the care of people who have cancer and in the education of oncologists and other health professionals who work with cancer patients and survivors.

ANCIENT WISDOM, MODERN SCIENCE

Mind-body approaches—chanting, imagery, hypnosis, dance, and relaxed deep breathing—are as old as the first aboriginal healing systems and as widespread as Chinese, Indian, African, and Native American medicine. It is only in the last 30 years, however, that modern Western medicine has begun to give these techniques the kind of importance they had in the first Western system of healing in Hippocratic-era Greece.

Mind-body approaches to healing are based on the understanding that our thoughts and feelings, and our beliefs and attitude, can affect and shape every aspect of our biologic functioning. Mind-body approaches also recognize that everything we do with our physical body—what we eat and how we stand, the ways we stretch our muscles and the tension that constricts them—can modify mental, psychologic, and physical functioning. Finally, mind-body approaches are based on the understanding that the mind and body are, in fact, inseparable, and that the central and peripheral nervous system, the endocrine and immune systems, all the organs of the body, and all the emotional responses we have share a common chemical language [1–3] and are constantly communicating with one another.

Ten years ago my students learned that mind-body therapies can make a difference to people who have cancer. Today, the clinical evidence is significantly stronger. These approaches offer an opportunity for patients who have cancer to participate actively in their own care. As the rapidly growing body of research tells us, these approaches have the promise to significantly reduce stress and enhance immunity, to enhance the quality of the lives of people who have cancer, and, perhaps, to increase the length of their survival.

The scientific frontiers of mind-body medicine were opened in three phases over the last century by pioneering researchers and clinicians who shared a capacity to see and appreciate the power of connections that other investigations had ignored. Walter Bradford Cannon [4], the great physiologist, paved the way for modern mind-body medicine at the beginning of the twentieth century. Cannon, who taught at Harvard, described the dynamic equilibrium, or balance of forces within an organism, as homeostasis (from the Greek *homoios*, meaning "similar," and *stasis*, meaning "position"). He also described patterns of behavior and physiology that were common to all the animals he studied, from mice to men. Among these was the response he named "fight or flight."

Cannon observed that all vertebrates had a coherent response to a threat, whether the danger was an oncoming storm or a marauding predator. The response included an increase in heart and respiratory rates, greater tension in large muscle groups, coldness and sweatiness, a decrease in intestinal activity, and a dilation of the pupils.

All these, Cannon noted, were manifestations of activity on the part of the sympathetic nervous system, one of two branches of the autonomic (beyond our control, as opposed to voluntary) nervous system. The sympathetic nervous system, like its complement, the parasympathetic nervous system, is regulated in the brain by the hypothalamus. It communicates not only with centers in the lungs, heart, and arteries but also with the adrenal medulla. There, it provokes the release of epinephrine and norepinephrine, which further stimulate heart and respiratory rates. All of this sympathetic activity, Cannon observed, primes animals—and humans—to flee from a predator or, if necessary, to fight.

The next major contribution to our understanding of the mind-body connection came in the 1920s and 1930s with the work of the Hungarian-born Canadian physician Hans Selye [5]. As a medical student in the 1920s, Selye had observed that people in the hospital all had a certain sick look about them, regardless of the diagnosis. As a researcher, he set himself the task of discovering whether there were consistent anatomic and physiologic changes in all these sick people, regardless of the particular illness each endured.

Selye pinched and poked animals and subjected them to heat and cold and loud noises, electrical shocks, and overcrowding. What he learned was that all animals, regardless of the nature of the noxious stimulus, and in addition to such local manifestations as bruises and burns, showed certain consistent responses. These included an enlargement of the adrenal cortex (which secretes steroid hormones, such as cortisol, that accelerate physiologic functioning and decrease inflammation) and shrinkage of the thymus, spleen, and lymph nodes, the major organs of the immune system. Selye [5] declared that all of these were responses to what he called "stress." He defined stress as "the non-specific response of the body to any demand" and the physiologic changes as "the general adaptation syndrome".

By the early 1970s, researchers were beginning to suggest that the fight-or-flight and stress responses might contribute to the onset of various human disease states. According to Cannon's observations, endangered animals quickly flee and quickly recover or else die fighting. Some "civilized" humans, however, seemed to later researchers to exist in a perpetual state of fight-or-flight. The angry, time-obsessed, hypertension and heart attack–prone "type A" executive, described by cardiologists Meyer Friedman and Ray Rosenman [6], was the prime example. Feeling unable either to fight or flee (he might lose his job or his status either way), hoping things would get better, toughing it out, the type A person was in a chronic state of anxious readiness. In time, Friedman and Rosenman hypothesized, this state produced physical damage, most significantly in the arteries and heart. Researchers now believe that repressed hostility is the primary culprit [7] in perpetuating the fight-or-flight response and in precipitating damage to the heart, but the basic principle—that prolonged fight-or-flight responses can cause disease—still holds.

Selye's work also suggested a physiologic basis for correlations that were being observed between early or ongoing emotional trauma—the loss of a parent or a spouse, for example, or chronic tension—and an increased incidence of cancer, depression, and other chronic illnesses. Clinicians and researchers suggested that perhaps people whose immune functioning was compromised by high levels of stress and prolonged secretion of steroids were more likely to exhibit the deficient immune response sometimes observed in cancer and the disordered immune functioning of autoimmune diseases (such as rheumatoid arthritis) and a vulnerability to chronic infections.

By the early 1970s it had occurred to clinicians and researchers that if stressful situations and stressed-out personalities were conducive to heart disease, cancer, and other illnesses, it was entirely plausible that decreasing stress and improving outlook might help prevent these illnesses, and, indeed, contribute to better treatment. This hypothesis would stimulate new studies on stress-related illness and new ways to deal with it. It would give energy and importance to the new fields of stress reduction, mind-body medicine, and psycho-oncology. Over the following 35 years this hypothesis would provide the impetus for millions of people around the world to explore a wide range of mind-body therapies.

At about the same time, other lines of research, initiated by George Solomon [8] at Stanford, Robert Ader and David Felten [9] at the University of Rochester, and Candace Pert and Solomon Snyder [2] at Johns Hopkins, were suggesting a third pathway by which mental attitudes and emotional responses could affect physical functioning and produce illness.

In the 1960s, Solomon, a psychiatrist, followed up on a little-known Soviet study that suggested that hypothalamus is the "headquarters" of immune regulation and the autonomic nervous and endocrine system of functioning. He found that when he destroyed the hypothalamus in rats, they exhibited a marked decline in immune functioning. Ten years later, Ader discovered that the cells of the immune system, which had always been regarded as an autonomous defense network, could in fact be conditioned in much the same way that the Russian physiologist Ivan Pavlov had conditioned dogs to salivate at the sound of a bell. Not long after, Ader's colleague, Felten, demonstrated direct connections between the fibers of the sympathetic nervous system and the organs and cells of the immune system. Meanwhile, Pert and Snyder were revealing that similar receptors for peptides exist on the walls of cells in the brain and the immune system.

Solomon pinpointed the central role of the hypothalamus in immunity. Ader [9] showed that the mind, presumably acting once again through the hypothalamus, could affect immune activity. Felten helped describe the physical connections that make this possible. Pert and Snyder [2] were suggesting another kind of connection and another mode of communication—peptide messengers—between the cells of the brain and those of the immune system. Ader [9] named the new field they were mapping psychoneuroimmunology, to emphasize the interconnections among the mind, brain, and immune system.

As this work accumulated, the connections between the mind and the emotions it produces and three of the body's most important regulatory systems—the autonomic nervous, endocrine, and immune systems—became ever clearer. A panoramic picture of the links among social stress and thoughts, feelings, and physical functioning began to emerge. It looked as if the kind of stress we experience, and the ways in which we interpret and deal with it, might be significant factors in the production of many of the diseases from which we suffer, as if stress might well contribute to the onset and course of cancer.

STRESS AS A CAUSE OF CANCER: WHAT DO WE KNOW?

For almost 2000 years, clinicians have observed that people who have cancer are more likely to be depressed or grief-stricken, lonely or overwhelmed, than those who do not have the disease—from the second century AD, when Galen had noted that women who had breast cancer were "melancholic," to the end of the nineteenth century, when the distinguished United States surgeon, William Parker, observed that grief is especially associated with all forms of cancer [10].

When the psychologist Claus Bahnson [11] reviewed the literature on stress, emotions, and cancer in 1980, he focused on a "particular configuration" in patients who had cancer, one "characterized by denial and depression" and absence or loss of affection in early childhood, "severe loss" in later life, and strong and persistent feelings of hopelessness and helplessness.

Bahnson had several recent studies to draw on: Caroline Thomas's [12] 30-year prospective study of Johns Hopkins medical students, which had revealed a correlation between "lack of closeness to parents and later occurrence of cancer"; Schmale and Spence's [11] observation that women who had suspicious cervical cancer biopsies who had recently suffered loss were more likely to subsequently develop cervical cancer; and Le Shan [13,14] and Worthington's findings that patients who had cancer were significantly more likely than controls to have "suffered loss of an important relationship" before their diagnosis and to "have no ability to express hostile feelings."

In the past 25 years, researchers have sought to confirm these findings and to use the new understanding of psychoneuroimmunology to correlate them with changes in immune functioning. It has become clear, for example, that stress of various kinds—from loss of a spouse to upcoming medical school examinations—can decrease immune functioning [15,16], lowering the number of natural killer cells (which seem to be involved in tumor surveillance), and impairing the effectiveness of DNA repair [17]. These findings suggest that stress can make us less capable of defending ourselves against the development of cancer by weakening our defenses against mutations and by rendering immune cells less competent.

More recent studies on personality and cancer have confirmed some, but not all, of the earlier work that Bahnson cited. It seems that certain kinds of people are somewhat more likely to develop cancer: those who have experienced prolonged stress, particularly stress from which they have been unable to escape [18]; those who have suffered significant losses early in life; and those who have what has been called a "repressive coping" style [19], a pronounced tendency to deny and repress their own feelings, which has been described as a "type C personality" [20].

These studies most emphatically do not mean that all people, or even a significant number of people, who have lost a parent at an early age or been under prolonged stress or are uncomfortable expressing feelings will develop cancer. The association or influence is, as the gifted researcher Bernard Fox has repeatedly pointed out, at best a weak one [21]. There are many other factors—genetic, environmental, and dietary among them—that probably play far larger roles in the development of cancer.

These studies on physiology and psychology do, however, suggest that all clinicians need to pay attention to the stresses in their patients' lives before and after the diagnosis of cancer. They encourage us to help all of our patients to deal with, rather than deny, the existence of situations in which they feel trapped, to express rather than repress their emotions, and to take action to help themselves rather than wait for others to take charge.

STRESS AFTER THE DIAGNOSIS OF CANCER

Several studies suggest that stress, particularly our attitudes toward it, may have far more impact on people after the diagnosis of cancer than before. For example, many studies show that quality of life [22]—how someone who has cancer feels physically and emotionally, how well he or she functions in the world, and the level of distress from cancer and its treatment—is an important factor in predicting not only how well but also how long someone who has cancer will live. That is, patients who have lung or breast cancer who are generally more optimistic and energetic, more involved in their usual activities, and more hopeful about their future are more likely to continue to feel better and may, indeed, live longer than if they feel less optimistic or less engaged—even if the type of cancer and its stage are identical [23,24].

These observations dovetailed with work of Steven Greer and colleagues [25–27] on stress and cancer survival. In several landmark studies, beginning in 1972, they established a relationship between coping styles and a more favorable outcome for patients who have cancer. They began by asking whether the psychologic stance that patients adopt when they develop cancer can, in some cases, influence the course of their disease. They interviewed a group of women who had breast cancer at the beginning of treatment and 3 months after diagnosis. All of the women had similar diagnoses—a stage II cancer, which had only spread to some of the surrounding breast tissue—and were treated with surgery and, in some cases, radiation.

Greer's study followed these patients for 15 years. The psychologic response—the coping style of the patient—was related to the disease outcome at 5 years, 10 years, and 15 years. The conclusions are striking. Recurrence-free survival was significantly more common in patients whose coping style was characterized by "fighting spirit" or "denial" than in patients who showed either "stoic acceptance" or "helplessness and hopelessness." At the final follow-up, 45% of the women who responded to a diagnosis of breast cancer with a fighting spirit or denial were alive and well with no evidence of recurrence, compared with 17% who exhibited other responses.

Using similar criteria in other studies, other researchers found that a coping style characterized as either stoic acceptance or helpless/hopeless led to faster progression of cancer in patients who had melanoma, cervical cancer, uterine and ovarian cancer, and (in men) the general incidence of cancer. More recently, a study by Greer's collaborators [28] showed that in another group of women who had breast cancer, helpless and hopeless coping styles did have a detrimental effect on survival but fighting spirit did not seem to improve longevity.

Some critics strongly question whether Greer's questionnaire is as valid today as it was in the 1970s, given the vast cultural changes in attitudes that have occurred about illness and cancer. Still, the bulk of these studies suggest that coping style can significantly affect the progression of cancer [20,29].

This work on attitude and coping is bolstered by studies on the effect of stress on the growth and progression of various kinds of tumors probably through dysregulation of the immune system [29,30]. Generally speaking, stress—particularly prolonged and major stress (this includes the stress of significant life events, such as loss of a job or spouse and, most definitely, of coping with the knowledge that one has cancer and with its treatment)—stimulates tumor growth. This effect seems to be mediated in part by higher levels of cortisol and adrenaline, which depress immune functioning and may promote tumor vascularization [31].

This finding makes intuitive sense. Cancer taxes our capacity to maintain physical homeostasis and emotional equilibrium in many significant ways. It may well make us more vulnerable to situations and stressors with which we previously would have dealt more easily.

On the other hand, knowing that all of us are vulnerable to stress and what is stressful to us can help us help our patients deal with it better. This observation is true because, ultimately, stress is a subjective experience. If you believe the job you may lose is the only one you will ever have, your level of stress is vastly different than if you are open to the possibility that losing this particular job may open the door for you to find another, better one. If people see themselves as helpless victims and cancer as an overwhelming enemy, they experience far more stress than if they believe they can do something to help themselves; if they see cancer as an opportunity to find out what really matters in their lives, if they see it as a challenge rather than simply a disaster, it makes sense that they feel less stress and deal with their disease more effectively [32,33].

The mind-body approach, and the techniques that it makes use of, can be central to transforming the meaning of cancer and to dealing effectively with the stress it inevitably brings. As people who have cancer use the techniques that are included in this approach, they begin to address their psychologic vulnerability to stress and its physiologic consequences. Each time patients practice any of the techniques described—relaxation, meditation, imagery, autogenic training, hypnosis, self-expression, and exercise—they experience specific physiologic benefits: decreases in stress; improvements in sleep, mood, and pain; a decrease in stress hormones; and enhanced immunity. Each time they feel the benefit of the technique they are using they reinforce their sense of control over their own lives and counter whatever feelings of hopelessness and helplessness they may feel.

All of these mind-body techniques are supported by scientific evidence and a physiologic rationale, but no technique is definitely proved "better" than the others. In deciding which technique or which combination of techniques to use, it is important to individualize them according to the needs and preferences of each patient [34]. You can understand the mind-body approach far better, and recommend it to your patients with more authentic authority, if you have experienced and made use of these techniques yourself. Standard therapeutic modalities (surgery, chemotherapy, radiation, and so forth) of course require intervention by a skilled professional. Mind-body approaches are a form of self-care. Knowing the research literature on them is valuable and will, I hope, encourage you to recommend them, but the authority with which you present them is vastly enhanced by your personal and professional experience of their therapeutic power.

MIND-BODY TECHNIQUES

Relaxation

Relaxation is the most basic of mind-body techniques and the precondition for successfully using many of the more complex interventions. It is also our birthright as humans. People in aboriginal or village cultures devote far more time to relaxation than do hyperactive modern men and women. Relaxation is a natural part of their lives, a long pause between activities, and often the attitude toward all activities they engage in. It is sad but true that most of us in the United States have to make a conscious effort to make relaxation a part of our lives, to remind ourselves of its importance, and to take time for it. When people have cancer they have to make even more of an effort to relax.

They need to accept the fear and apprehension that so often accompany a diagnosis and by doing so, soften its impact. They also have to begin in the face of fear and frustration, by trying to relax.

Physiologically, relaxation means a reduction in the sympathetic nervous system excitation that marks the fight-or-flight response and a decrease in the level of stress. According to almost 40 years of research, much of it done by Herbert Benson [35] and his colleagues at the Mind-Body Medical Institute at Harvard Medical School, relaxation can be powerful medicine: A small quantity can produce significant results. Relaxing 15 or 20 minutes, twice a day, can lower levels of adrenaline and cortisol; decrease blood pressure, heart rate, and respiration; enhance immune functioning; and balance the activity in the right and left hemispheres of the brain.

Regular relaxation has yielded impressive results for people who have cancer: decreased levels of stress and increased immune functioning [36]; decreased pain [37]; fewer side effects from chemotherapy [38]; and decreased anxiety, improved mood, and less suppression of emotions [39]. Generally speaking, brief use of relaxation has only short-term effects, whereas ongoing practice throughout and beyond the course of conventional treatment is likely to produce more lasting benefits [40–42].

In our mind-body skills groups at The Center for Mind-Body Medicine we begin with a simple, slow deep-breathing technique called "soft belly" (Box 1) that you can use yourself and teach to your patients. Soft belly is just one of many forms of relaxation. There is an almost infinite variety of techniques that can be used: the repetition of a religious phrase or an ordinary word that is meaningful to the individual; a prayer or a word, such as "one"; or quiet

---

Box 1: Soft belly breathing

In our mind-body skills groups at The Center for Mind-Body Medicine we begin with a simple technique, soft belly, that you can use yourself and teach to your patient. Here are the instructions:

- Close your eyes, breathe deeply, in through the nose and out through the mouth.
- Imagine your belly is soft; this deepens the breath and improves the exchange of oxygen, even as it relaxes your muscles.
- Say to yourself "soft" as you breathe in and "belly" as you breathe out.
- We suggest that our group members continue this approach for 5 or 10 minutes. Each day they add another minute or two to it.
- Do this two or three times a day—not right after meals, you may fall asleep—and at bedtime, if you are having trouble sleeping.
- Use a timer (but not at bedtime) so you are not preoccupied with how long you've been doing it or how long you have left.
- Soon, you'll find that in times of stress you can take a few deep breaths and say, "Soft...belly," and relaxation will come.

repetitive activity. Several studies have also shown that relaxation techniques can be successfully paired with and perhaps enhanced by music [43–46]. The technique simply needs to be one that is relaxing for you.

Relaxation also helps people who have cancer to gain perspective on every aspect of their lives and to feel less overwhelmed by the challenges of cancer and its treatment. If people who have cancer can relax during a difficult time, it becomes, by definition, no longer such a powerful stressor to them.

Meditation

Meditation is a combination of relaxation and self-awareness. Although it is normally thought of as synonymous with a particular technique, meditation is, in fact, an attitude and a way of life, a relaxed awareness of all that arises in our lives and in our minds, of our thoughts, feelings, and sensations. Meditation comes from the same Sanskrit word as medicine, a word that means "to take the measure of" and "to care for." Meditation is a technique for bringing us into the present moment and the experience of living in that moment, free from anxiety about the past or apprehension about the future.

There are three basic kinds of meditation. The first, "concentrative" meditation, focuses on a particular phrase or sound (as in the Sanskrit mantra, or sound, "om") or a visual image (a candle or picture). The soft belly exercise described previously is a relaxation technique and a form of concentrative meditation.

The second kind is "awareness" or "mindfulness" meditation. Its prototype is a South Asian Buddhist form called Vipassana. In awareness meditation one simply becomes aware of thoughts, feelings, and sensations as they arise. You can do awareness meditation sitting or walking, or bring awareness to any activity: cooking, cleaning, eating, ordinary office tasks, caring for a child, making love, or even experiencing chemotherapy.

The third form is "expressive" meditation. This form includes fast deep breathing, shaking, whirling, and dancing—techniques that move the body and evoke, energize, and release emotions. This is the oldest form of meditation and is still practiced in many tribal societies.

Most of the early research that was done on meditation and cancer focused on concentrative meditations but was usually characterized as relaxation. More recently there have been some impressive studies on the usefulness of mindfulness mediation [47–51]. One follow-up study for patients who had breast and prostate cancer that combined guided imagery and the postures of Hatha yoga in a group setting in which mindfulness was emphasized and practiced produced "altered cortisol and immune patterns... consistent with less stress and mood disturbance" as well as enhanced quality of life and decreased symptoms of stress [52].

There is no research on expressive meditation, although many patients we have worked with at The Center for Mind-Body Medicine have found shaking while standing for several minutes, followed by dancing, both energizing and relaxing. All forms of meditation help patients feel the mind-body connection.

Expressive meditation also offers a pleasurable experience of one's body, which is particularly important during and after treatments that may have brought with them pain, discomfort, and a negatively altered body image.

Imagery

Imagery is almost certainly the mind-body technique most widely and happily used by people who have cancer, with good reason. Imagery is an innate skill that all of us seem to possess. We all know the pleasure of daydreaming or removing ourselves from an unpleasant situation by letting our minds wander and the exhilaration of imagining things exactly as we want. The practice of guided imagery makes use of this human capacity in a directed and powerfully therapeutic way.

Jeanne Achterberg [53], who did some of the first research on the therapeutic effects of imagery with patients who have cancer, defines imagery as "the thought process that evokes and uses the senses...[I]t is the communication mechanism between perception, emotion and bodily change". Imagery includes auditory, kinesthetic, and gustatory images—those of sound and bodily feeling and taste—and visual images. It stimulates specific areas of our brain as effectively as if we were actually seeing, or hearing, or tasting [54,55].

There are two basic kinds of imagery techniques [56]. Receptive imagery is the use of relaxed meditative state to access information from what we sometimes call the unconscious, or our intuition. Active imagery involves actively imaging some desired result. Both have practical uses for people who have cancer.

Active imagery, which is most often used in clinical settings, involves the conscious, directed use of the imagination to activate a healing response. This kind of imagery was first popularized 35 years ago by radiation oncologist Carl Simonton and psychologist Stephanie Matthews Simonton [57]. The Simontons encouraged images of immune cells conquering or obliterating cancer cells as, for example, powerful, handsome knights on white horses slaying creepy-looking, ill-equipped armies of cancer cells. In her early studies of the Simontons' work, Achterberg showed that people who had cancer who spontaneously had these kinds of powerful—even aggressive—images had a better prognosis than those who spontaneously came up with images in which, for example, the cancer cells were overwhelming the white blood cells [53,58].

In the years since then, it has become increasingly clear how individualized imagery is. Not everyone wants to or is served by envisioning a battle in which white blood cells destroy cancer cells. The kinds of images that are most effective vary from person to person. For example, some people prefer anatomically correct images of white blood cells and cancer cells. Others prefer images that are metaphoric, such as a big broom sweeping up cancer cells. Some people feel empowered by the Simontons' warlike images, but others prefer quieter images: cancer cells fading in smoke or packing up and leaving the body.

Most of the published research on imagery has been on various kinds of active imagery. Sometimes, the studies compare guided imagery to relaxation. In some of them, the combination of guided imagery and relaxation is more effective than relaxation by itself [36,38,39]. The effects of relaxation and guided imagery are often hard to tease apart—even soft belly is an image. What is important from a practical perspective, however, is that the overwhelming majority of studies show that the combination of relaxation and imagery is helpful for pain control [37,59–62], recovery from cancer surgery [63], decreasing the nausea and vomiting of chemotherapy [38,63–65] and the distress of radiation [66,67], facilitating emotional expression and enhancing quality of life [61,68], and increasing the production and functioning of immune cells, including T cells and natural killer cells [65,69,70].

Hypnosis

Hypnosis is defined as a combination of relaxation, suggestion, and focused attention. It can be understood as a specific way of inducing relaxation and directing guided imagery. Some hypnotherapists who work with patients who have cancer, such as Bernauer Newton [71], have emphasized the profound state of relaxation that hypnosis can induce. Newton regards this as the medium in which the body can restore homeostasis. Others focus on the ways in which specific hypnotic suggestions may be used, like images, to focus on decreasing pain or enhancing immune response.

It is difficult and, ultimately, not important to distinguish between hypnosis and imagery. What is important is that hypnosis, like imagery, makes use of the mind's extraordinary power to affect physical functioning.

Research on hypnotic techniques overlaps with, and is at least as impressive as, the research on imagery. As the studies published in peer-reviewed journals have shown, hypnotic techniques can be used in various ways for people who have cancer [72]: to reduce severe pain by 50% or more [73–75], to decrease nausea and vomiting in patients undergoing chemotherapy [76–78], to decrease anxiety and enhance quality of life [72,76,79], and to facilitate pain-free procedures [80].

Hypnosis has been found to be of particular help to children who in general find mind-body approaches extremely easy to learn and use. Studies [75] have repeatedly shown its effectiveness in reducing the pain that accompanies procedures, in decreasing the nausea and vomiting produced by chemotherapy, and in decreasing anxiety.

Biofeedback and Autogenic Training

In 1961, when Neal Miller [81] first suggested that the autonomic nervous system could be as susceptible to training as the voluntary nervous system, that we might learn to control our heart rate and our bowel contractions just as we learned to walk or type or play tennis, his audiences were aghast. He was a respected researcher, director of a laboratory at Yale, but this was a kind of scientific heresy. Everyone knew that the autonomic nervous system was precisely that—autonomic, beyond our control. The fabled feats of Indian yogis—their claimed ability to slow the rate of their heart and their breathing and to profoundly alter their body temperature—were regarded at that time as a masochist's perversion, a charlatan's tricks, or neurologic accidents.

Miller persisted. He was convinced that the difference between the autonomic and voluntary nervous systems was not so much one of kind but of opportunity. The skeletal system is subject to visible and immediate correction from the environment: seeing the disastrous results of your looping tennis forehand encourages and enables you to shorten your swing. The results of the autonomic nervous system's actions are not immediately apparent. We do not see or feel or hear anything when our blood pressure increases.

Miller believed, and soon proved, that if he simply offered a perceptible recording of autonomic behavior—sounding a high-pitched tone, for example, until elevated blood pressure decreased or cold hands warmed—people would be able to use this information to correct internal functioning. This procedure, which Miller first demonstrated in dogs and in rats, by teaching them to salivate both more and less and to raise and lower their heart rates, is biofeedback.

Biofeedback worked. People learned to use it to lower blood pressure and to increase hand temperature. Soon enough, clinicians began to use it for common and debilitating problems. For example, because the arterial constriction that is prominent in the first phase of migraine headaches also causes cold hands, feedback of information about finger temperature can be used as a form of treatment of migraines: the patient who learns to increase the temperature in his or her hands by relaxing the muscular walls of the blood vessels there is automatically doing the same thing with the blood vessels in the head.

Over the last 30 years, physicians, psychologists, and biofeedback technicians, in tandem with engineers, have developed sensors and procedures that have enabled hundreds of thousands of people to become aware of and to control even the most obscure aspects of their physiologic functioning [82,83]. For example, patients can now use readouts of tension from their urethral and anal sphincters to control urinary and fecal incontinence, conditions that often resist all other medical and surgical interventions. This application can be particularly important for postprostatectomy patients who have incontinence [84]. Biofeedback of various kinds also has wider applications for patients who have cancer, including pain relief [85,86], relieving side effects of chemotherapy [87], and inducing sleep and reducing stress [85,88].

Biofeedback not only produces replicable and powerful changes in physiology and improvement in symptoms but it also gives patients who have cancer a sense of connection to and control over their internal processes. This sense of mastery often generalizes to other aspects of their lives: people who have practiced biofeedback for a specific condition find it far easier to induce a relaxed state when confronted with any kind of stress. In time, many people who use biofeedback monitors learn to effect the same kinds of changes without them, using the power of their minds alone.

Autogenic training, which is sometimes paired with biofeedback, can also be used on its own. Although it is not well known in the United States, autogenic training, which was developed by German neurologist Johannes Schultz in the

1930s, is one of the simplest, most widely used, and best-researched forms of self-hypnosis. Making use of a sequence of seven phrases that describe bodily feelings and encourage parasympathetic nervous system activity ("my arms are warm and heavy," "my legs are warm and heavy," and so on) it is sometimes used as a prelude to biofeedback. It is also capable of inducing deep states of relaxation and relieving various physical symptoms, including those associated with cancer and its treatment [89,90].

Self-Expression

Self expression—through words, artwork, and movement—is an important anti-dote to the feelings of helplessness and hopelessness that beset so many people who have cancer [91].

Psychologist James Pennebaker [92–94] and his colleagues have shown that writing about stressful events—expressing rather than repressing feelings about them—can enhance well-being, reduce emotional stress, decrease frequency of medical visits, and even improve immune functioning. Published studies have demonstrated the effects of this kind of self-expression in people who have suffered emotional trauma and on patients who have rheumatoid arthritis and asthma [95].

In the research studies, people are generally asked to write about traumatic events for 20 minutes or more, on each of three successive days. Cancer and its diagnosis would, of course, qualify as traumatic, and so too would any other events that were or are deeply disturbing: loss of a parent, a spouse, or a rela-tionship; accidents; terrible disappointments at work; and side effects and set-backs in cancer treatment. There are now specific studies on the benefits of verbal expression for people who have cancer [96,97].

Humor is an aspect of self-expression that may be particularly helpful. It pro-vides relief from and gives patients perspective on their ongoing, serious, and often fearful preoccupations with cancer and its treatment. Published studies reviewed by Christie [98] have shown increases in feelings of well-being and enhanced coping and decreases in stress hormones in various healthy and chronically ill populations. One study [99] shows the positive effect of humor on women dealing with the breast cancer diagnosis. Another study [100] of par-ticular relevance to oncology professionals reveals the importance of humor in relieving stress among nurses, house staff, and medical oncologists who work daily with patients who have cancer.

Art Therapy

Drawings and art therapy have long been used as a way for children who have cancer to express and deal more productively with the troubled and fearful thoughts, frightening feelings [101,102], and physical pain [103] that cancer and its treatment may evoke. In recent years, the benefits of this approach have been extended to adults, particularly to women who have breast cancer [104–106]. Although many of these interventions have been undertaken by fully trained art therapists, other clinicians can use simple, easily learned drawing techniques to encourage self-expression, reduce pain, and promote positive coping strategies.

Exercise

Physical exercise is often hard for patients who have cancer to imagine, let alone do. They may feel exhausted from treatment and more frail than ever before. The bodies that once gave them pleasure may now seem like a burden. They may wonder, too, why their oncologists have not encouraged them to exercise. These can be obstacles, but they are not insurmountable ones.

Exercise (Box 2) should be regarded by oncology professionals and patients who have cancer as a central element of any program of integrative and comprehensive care. At this point, the research literature, which was sparse when my students examined it 10 years ago, is robust [107,108]. Exercise, it seems, can make significant contributions to the reduction of treatment-associated side effects [109–113], to relieving the fatigue that often bedevils patients who have cancer [114,115], and especially to enhancing quality of life and mood [107,108,111,116–121]. Exercise also seems to help prevent the occurrence of cancer [122–127] and may therefore have a role in preventing recurrence. Exercise also helps people who have cancer who experience their bodies as a source of distress and embarrassment to rediscover pleasure and satisfaction in them.

One form of exercise—the postures and breathing techniques of Hatha yoga—has recently received increasing and deserved attention [128–132]. A recent study conducted with a largely African American and Hispanic group of patients who had breast cancer [133] showed significant improvements in quality of life, enhanced emotional and social well-being, and less distracted mood, as these patients practiced regularly.

Yoga is particularly promising because it is often more accessible than other exercise to people who feel debilitated by cancer and its treatment, and because it promotes a more meditative and relaxed attitude toward all the challenges that cancer brings.

Box 2: Summary: these mind-body techniques have significant scientific support for use with people who have cancer

- Relaxation
- Meditation
- Guided imagery
- Hypnosis
- Biofeedback and autogenic training
- Self-expression in words
- Art and music therapy
- Exercise and yoga

SOCIAL SUPPORT

In traditional societies, the official healers—shamans, witch doctors, and wise women—who deal with life-threatening illness understand that these conditions represent an imbalance in the social order and in the body of the affected individual. Healing involves not only the herbs and advice that are the province of the indigenous professional, but also bringing the extended family or the village together in rituals to restore the social balance. These ceremonies purge social dysfunction and re-establish communal connections, the soil that these cultures believe nurtures all other healing.

In recent years we in the industrialized West have slowly begun to recover this wisdom. Increasingly, epidemiologic studies and clinical research have helped us to appreciate the power of human connections and of social context generally, in contributing to, preventing, and treating our most serious illness including, most particularly, cancer. Epidemiologic studies have informed us that mortality rates are consistently higher among the unmarried than the married and that unmarried, socially isolated individuals have higher rates of infectious disease, accidents, and suicides. The landmark multiyear study of residents of Alameda County, California revealed that the mortality rates for the most socially isolated men were 2.3 times as great as for those who had the most social contacts and that for women the differential was even greater [134].

Various factors may contribute to these findings—for example, our understanding that poor diet and less regular general health habits are more common among more isolated people. That much, but by no means all, of the data on people who have cancer (see later discussion) come from studies on women may have some significance also. Perhaps, in our society, women appreciate and thrive on social connections more than men. The trend is clear that isolation makes us more vulnerable to chronic illness, including cancer; human connections help us to heal.

Research, particularly that done by Janice Kiecolt-Glaser and her colleagues [94,135,136], has suggested that isolation depresses immune functioning and that group support mitigates this effect.

The studies on the impact of social support on people who have already been diagnosed with cancer are even more dramatic. These studies indicate that people who have various cancers who have a higher degree of social involvement—more friends and relatives whom they see, greater participation in religious and other community groups—have a better quality of life and may tend to live longer. One of these studies, by the Canadian epidemiologist Elizabeth Maunsell [137], was published in *Cancer* in 1995. Women who had breast cancer (confined to the breast or local lymph nodes) who had no confidants had a 7-year survival rate of 56%, whereas those who had two or more confidants had a survival rate of 76%.

WHAT ABOUT SUPPORT GROUPS?

In the past 20 years the numbers and types of support groups for people who have cancer have grown exponentially. There are groups that provide practical advice—some that deal with chemotherapy and radiation, colostomies, and ileostomies—and groups that are concerned with spirituality and prayer [138–141]. There are groups that are open to anyone who has cancer and those confined to people who have brain tumors or prostate cancer; groups for adults and for children; large, classroomlike, drop-in groups whose membership fluctuates significantly from session to session, and closed groups with a fixed membership; groups that meet for a specific period of time and groups that may go on for years; groups with professional leaders, and those in which the leadership role may rotate from patient to patient.

Most of the research that has been done is on small, closed, professionally led, time-limited, intimate, and focused groups. Stanford University psychiatrist David Spiegel [142,143] created such a group for women who had metastatic breast cancer in 1976. He defined these groups as "supportive/expressive," meaning that the women in them had the opportunity to share with one another what they were feeling and thinking. The groups were led by Spiegel and other psychiatrists and met once a week for an hour and a half for a year. The women in them learned some relaxation exercises and self-hypnosis to control pain and discomfort. They were also encouraged to talk about what was going on in their lives, in and out of treatment, and about the possibility of death.

The research Spiegel did was carefully controlled. All 86 women received the best conventional medical treatment at Stanford University Hospital. Fifty of them were in support groups; 36 served as controls. Spiegel found that the women in the groups came to care deeply about one another; they helped each other formulate questions for their doctors and sometimes even accompanied one another to appointments. When a group member died, they mourned together.

Spiegel had organized the groups expecting an improvement in the quality of life for the women who participated in them. Early results after the last session showed that the women were, as predicted, "less anxious and depressed and were coping more effectively with breast cancer" [142]. The study was a success and suggested that support groups were an important tool.

Ten years after the groups ended, Spiegel did a follow-up study. He was astonished to find that the women in the support groups had lived twice as long as the controls. He doubted his own data but the finding held and the landmark study "The Effect of Psychosocial Treatment on Survival of Patients with Metastatic Breast Cancer" was published in *Lancet* in 1989 [143]. This evidence made it clear that participation in a support group might contribute not only to emotional well-being but also to longevity.

Another study done at the University of California at Los Angeles by psychiatrist Fawzy and his colleagues [144] confirmed that support groups may significantly prolong the lives of patients who have cancer. In this study, patients who had melanoma met with a leader in small groups once a week for an hour and a half for 6 weeks. These patients received some education about their disease, learned a few relaxation techniques, did some work on problem solving, were given some assertiveness training, and had a chance to share their concerns with one another.

Six months after the study ended, the patients in the group had significantly better natural killer cell activity than those who received only conventional medical treatment. Six years later, group members had a significantly lower rate of tumor recurrence (21% versus 38%) and a dramatically lower death rate (9% versus 29%) [145,146].

Finally, a study by Jeanne Richardson [147] of patients who had leukemia and lymphoma demonstrated that patients who participated in a modest behavioral and educational home intervention lived significantly longer than those who did not. There was a 39% reduction in the rate of death.

Several other studies on the small-group interventions have not confirmed the striking findings of Spiegel, Fawzy, and Richardson. (In two of these negative studies, there was no significant improvement in psychologic status or longevity; the patients in the third study had very advanced cancers and no improvement.) In a large-scale attempt to replicate Spiegel's study in the United States and Canada, Goodwin and her colleagues [148] showed significantly improved quality of life but no increase in longevity. Most recently, in a second study Spiegel [149] himself did not find increased longevity in patients who had breast cancer treated with supportive-expressive group therapy.

The disparity between Spiegel's and Goodwin's results was striking and oncology professionals generally concluded that although support groups do not increase life span, they are valuable adjuncts to cancer care, generally decreasing levels of stress and enhancing quality of life and coping skills. The work of Alastair Cunningham [150–152] suggests another possible explanation for the disparity.

For many years, Cunningham and his colleagues led support groups at Princess Elizabeth Hospital in Ontario, Canada. These groups used many of the techniques described in this article, including meditation, guided imagery, and various introspective and expressive therapies—far more than in Spiegel's or Goodwin's groups. They also used them in a context that promoted psychologic and spiritual exploration and growth.

When Cunningham [152] aggregated the data on his patients who had advanced cancer and compared them to matched controls, he discovered no significant difference in longevity. When, however, he looked at a subset of patients who did live significantly longer, he discovered a clear pattern. These people had attended the groups regularly (as did Spiegel's and Goodwin's patients). They also made the practices taught a regular part of their daily life and used the lessons learned about the possibility of hope, meaning, and purpose, and their own capacity to reduce symptoms and enhance coping, as guiding principles in their lives.

Although the numbers were small, I believe the implications are significant. Support groups are not alike and membership by itself does not assure a life-changing or life-extending outcome; however, groups that offer patients various mind-body approaches to deal with their disease and provide them with an opportunity for self-discovery and a chance to see cancer as a life-challenging opportunity as well as a life-threatening disease may be particularly helpful, even extending life. This important therapeutic possibility needs to be studied in far more depth.

LOOKING AHEAD: LESSONS FOR PRACTICE

Over the last 35 years, it has become abundantly clear that mind-body approaches should be integrated into all cancer care. Although the level of evidence for the efficacy of the various techniques varies, and although it is sometimes difficult to distinguish which aspect of each technique is most effective (as I have noted, relaxation is integral to many of them and guided imagery and hypnosis are virtually indistinguishable), certain conclusions and guidelines seem justified.

- All oncology professionals, and all those who work with patients who have cancer, need to be informed about mind-body techniques and to experience them and prescribe them.
- Mind-body approaches can be helpful throughout the entire cancer experience, from the day of the anxiety-producing diagnosis through the end of conventional treatment and beyond; before, during, and after painful and interventions, including surgery, chemotherapy, and radiation; as a tool for dealing with the anxiety that cancer provokes; and as a practical way of enhancing coping skills.
- Mind-body techniques directly address the sense of hopelessness and helplessness that is particularly devastating to patients who have cancer. Their practice reinforces a sense of control and mastery.
- Many of these techniques, particularly expressive ones, such as dance, and physical exercise and yoga, may also help restore a sense of physical pleasure and satisfaction in people whose bodies have been damaged by cancer and its treatment.
- Groups, in which many of these therapies have been studied, are probably the best context for learning and practicing these mind-body and expressive techniques and also provide a source of support which is itself helpful and healing.
- The use of mind-body approaches and the way they are combined needs to be individualized for each patient.
- Creating a context in which mind-body approaches are encouraged as a way of life and a source of meaning and purpose may yield particularly significant therapeutic results.

References

[1] Pert C, Dienstfrey H. The neuropeptide network. Ann N Y Acad Sci 1998;521.
[2] Pert C. Molecules of emotion. New York: Scribner; 1997.
[3] Maier SF, Watkins LR. Cytokines for psychologists: implications of bidirectional immune-to-brain communication for understanding behavior, mood and cognition. Psychol Rev 1998;105(1):83–107.
[4] Cannon WB. The wisdom of the body. New York: W.W. Norton; 1926.
[5] Selye H. The stress of life. New York: McGraw-Hill; 1956.

[6] Freidman M, Rosenman RH. Type A behavior and your heart. New York: Knopf; 1974.

[7] Williams R. The trusting heart. New York: Times Books; 1989.

[8] Solomon GF. Emotions, immunity and disease. In: Temoshok L, et al, editors. Emotion in health and illness. New York: Times Books; 1989.

[9] Ader R, Felten DL, Cohen N, editors. Psychoneuroimmunology. 2nd edtion. San Diego (CA): Academic Press; 1991.

[10] Gordon JS, Curtin S. Comprehensive Cancer Care: Integrating Alternative, Complementary and Conventional Therapies. Cambridge: Perseus Books Group: Cambridge; May 30, 2000.

[11] Bahnson CB. Stress and cancer: the state of the art. Psychosomatics 1980;21(12):975.

[12] Thomas CB, Duszynski KR. Closeness to parents and the family constellation in a prospective study of five disease states: suicide, mental illness, malignant tumor, hypertension, and coronary heart disease. Johns Hopkins Med J 1974;134:251–70.

[13] LeShan L. Cancer as a turning point. Revised edition. New York: Penguin Group; 1994.

[14] LeShan L. A new question in studying psychosocial interventions and cancer. J Pers Soc Psychol 1991;61:899–909.

[15] Jemmott JB, Borysenko JZ, Borysenko M, et al. Academic stress, power motivation, and decrease in secretion rate of salivary secretory immunolobin a. Lancet 1983;25:1400–2.

[16] Pike JL, Smith TL, Hauger RL, et al. Chronic life stress alters sympathetic, neuroendocrine, and immune responsivity to an acute psychological stressor in humans. Psychosom Med 1997;59(4):447–57.

[17] Kiecolt-Glaser JK, Stephens RE, Lipetz PD, et al. Distress and DNA repair in human lymphocytes. J Behav Med 1985;l89(4):311–20.

[18] Laudenslager ML. Coping and immunosuppression: inescapable but not escapable shock suppresses lymphocyte proliferation. Science 1983;221:568–70.

[19] Greer S, Watson M. Towards a psychobiological model of cancer: psychological considerations. Soc Sci Med 1985;20(8):773–7.

[20] Temoshok L. Personality, coping style, emotion and cancer: towards an integrative model. Cancer Surv 1987;6(3):545–67.

[21] McKenna MC, Zevon MA, Corn B, Rounds J. Psychosocial factors and the development of breast cancer: a meta-analysis. Health Psychol 1999;18(5):52–61.

[22] Buccheri GF, Ferrigno D, Tamburnini M, et al. The patient's perception of his own quality of life might have an adjunctive prognostic significance in lung cancer. Lung Cancer 1995;12(1–2):45–58.

[23] Coates A, Gebsk V, Signorini D, et al. Prognostic value of quality of life scores during chemotherapy for advanced breast cancer. J Clin Oncol 1992;10(1):833–8.

[24] Ganz PA, Kee JJ, Diau J. Quality of life assessment: an independent prognostic variable for survival in lung cancer. Cancer 1991;67(3):131–5.

[25] Greer S. Psychological response to cancer and survival. Psychol Med 1991;21:43–9.

[26] Greer S. Mind-body research in psychooncology. Adv Mind Body Med 1999;15: 236–44.

[27] Greer S, Morris T, Pettingale KW, Haybittle JL. Psychological response to breast cancer and 15-year outcome. Lancet 1990;335:49–50.

[28] Watson M, Haviland JS, Greer S, Davidson J, Bliss JM. Influence of psychological response on survival in breast cancer: a population-based cohort study. Lancet 1999;354:1331–6.

[29] Sapolsky RM, Donnelly TM. Vulnerability to stress-induced tumor growth increases with age in rats: role of glucocorticoids. Endocrinology 1985;117(2):662–6.

[30] Marshall GD. Neuroendocrine mechanisms of immune dysregulation: applications to allergy and asthma. Ann Allergy Asthma Immunol 2004;93(2 Suppl 1):S11–7.

[31] Thaker PH, Han LY, Kamat AA, et al. Chronic stress promotes tumor growth and angiogenesis in a mouse model of ovarian carcinoma. Nat Med 2006;12(8):939–44.

[32] Spiegel D. Embodying the mind in psychooncology research. Adv Mind Body Med 1999;15:267–71.

[33] Folkman S. Thoughts about psychological factors, PNI, and cancer. Adv Mind Body Med 1999;15:255–9.

[34] Gruzelier JH. A review of the impact of hypnosis, relaxation, guided imagery and individual differences on aspects of immunity and health. Stress 2002;5(2):147–63.

[35] Benson H, Klipper MZ. The relaxation response. New York: William Morrow and Company; 1975.

[36] Bridge LR, Benson P, Pietroni PC, Priest RG. Relaxation and imagery in the treatment of breast cancer. BMJ 1988;297:1169–72.

[37] Syrjala KL, Donaldson GW, Davis MW, Kippes ME, Carr JE. Relaxation and imagery and cognitive-behavioral training reduce pain during cancer treatment: a controlled clinical trial. Pain 1995;63:189–98.

[38] Lyles JN, Burish TG, Krozely MG, Oldham RK. Efficacy of relaxation training and guided imagery in reducing the aversiveness of cancer chemotherapy. J Consult Clin Psychol 1982;50(4):509–24.

[39] Wallace KG. Analysis of recent literature concerning relaxation and imagery interventions for cancer pain. Cancer Nurs 1997;20(2):79–87.

[40] Campos de Carvalho E, Martins FT, dos Santos CB. A pilot study of a relaxation technique for management of nausea and vomiting in patients receiving cancer chemotherapy. Cancer Nurs 2007;30(2):163–7.

[41] Krischer MM, Xu P, Meade CD, et al. Self-administered stress management training in patients undergoing radiotherapy. J Clin Oncol 2007;25(29):4657–62.

[42] Anderson KO, Cohen MZ, Mendoza TR, et al. Brief cognitive-behavioral audiotape interventions for cancer-related pain. Cancer 2006;107(1):207–14.

[43] Burns DS, Sledge RB, Fuller LA, Daggy JK, Monahan PO. Cancer patients' interest and preferences for music therapy. J Music Ther 2005;42(3):185–99.

[44] Cassileth BR, Vickers AJ. Music therapy for mood disturbance during hospitalization for autologous stem cell transplantation. Cancer 2003;98(12):2723–30.

[45] Hillard RE. The effects of music therapy on the quality and length of life of people diagnosed with terminal cancer. J Music Ther 2003;40(2):113–37.

[46] Kwekkeboom KL. Music versus distraction for procedural pain and anxiety in patients with cancer. Oncol Nurs Forum 2003;30(3):433–40.

[47] Carlson LE, Speca M, Patel KD, Goodey E. Mindfulness-based stress reduction in relation to quality of life, mood, symptoms of stress, and immune parameters in breast and prostate cancer outpatients. Psychosom Med 2003;65(4):571–81.

[48] Carlson LE, et al. Mindfulness-based stress reduction in relation to quality of life, mood, symptoms of stress, and immune parameters in breast and prostate cancer outpatients. Psychosom Med 2003;65(4):571–81.

[49] Ott MJ, Speca M, Patel KD, Goodey E. Mindfulness meditation for oncology patients: a discussion and critical review. Integr Cancer Ther 2006;5(2):98–108.

[50] Shapiro SL, Bootzin RR, Figueredo AJ, Lopez AM, Schwartz GE. The efficacy of mindfulness-based stress reduction in the treatment of sleep disturbances in women with breast cancer. J Psychosom Res 2003;54:85–91.

[51] Smith JE, Richardson J, Hoffman C, et al. Mindfulness-based stress reduction as supportive therapy in cancer care: systematic review. J Adv Nurs 2005;52(3):315–27.

[52] Carlson LE, Speca M, Faris P, et al. One year pre-post intervention follow-up of psychological, immune, endocrine and blood pressure outcomes of mindfulness-based stress reduction (MBSR) in breast and prostate cancer outpatients. Brain Behav Immun 2007;21:1038–49.

[53] Information presented by Achterberg can be found in the 1998 Comprehensive Cancer Care (CCC) conference transcripts titled, "Imagery and Cancer Treatment," in the 1999 CCC transcripts titled, "Imagery and Cancer Treatment, and in the 1999 CCC workshop titled, "Covering CAM Therapies in the Journals". Available at: www.cmbm.org. Accessed 1999.

[54] Jeannerod M, Frak V. Mental imaging of motor activity in humans. Curr Opin Neurobiol 1999;9:735–9.

[55] Lotze M, Montoya P, Erb M, et al. Activation of cortical and cerebellar motor areas during executed and imagined hand movements: an fMRI study. J Cogn Neurosci 1999;11(5): 491–501.

[56] Achterberg J. Imagery in healing: shamanism and modern medicine. Boston: New Science Library, Shambala; 1985. p. 188–9.

[57] Simonton OC, Mathews-Simonton S, Creighton J. Getting well again. Los Angeles: J.P. Tracher; 1978.

[58] Donaldson VW. A clinical study of visualization on depressed white blood cell count in medical patients. Appl Psychophysiol Biofeedback 2000;25(2):117–28.

[59] Lewandowski W, Good M, Draucker CB. Changes in the meaning of pain with the use of guided imagery. Pain Manag Nurs 2005;6:58–67.

[60] Sloman R, Brown P, Aldana E, et al. The use of relaxation for the promotion of comfort and pain relief in persons with advanced cancer. Contemp Nurse 1995;3:6–12.

[61] Astin JA. Mind-body therapies for the management of pain. Clin J Pain 2004;20(1): 27–32.

[62] Huth MM, Broome ME, Good M. Imagery reduces children's post-operative pain. Pain 2004;110:439–48.

[63] Haase O, Schwenk W, Hermann C. Guided imagery and relaxation in conventional colorectal resections: a randomized, controlled, partially blinded trial. Dis Colon Rectum 2005;48:1955–63.

[64] Wyatt G, Sikorskii A, Siddii A. Feasibility of a reflexology and guided imagery intervention during chemotherapy: results of a quasi-experimental study. Oncol Nurs Forum 2007;34(3):635–42.

[65] Walker LG, Walker MB, Ogston K, et al. Psychological, clinical and pathological effects of relaxation training and guided imagery during primary chemotherapy. Br J Cancer 1999;80(1–2):262–8.

[66] Kolcaba K, Fox C. The effects of guided imagery on comfort of women with early stage breast cancer undergoing radiation therapy. Oncol Nurs Forum 1999;26(1): 67–72.

[67] Nunes DF, Rodriguez AL, da Silva Hoffmann F, et al. Relaxation and guided imagery program in patients with breast cancer undergoing radiotherapy is not associated with neuroimmunomodulatory effects. J Psychosom Res 2007;63:647–55.

[68] Ahn SH, Han OS, Kim SB, et al. Efficacy of progressive muscle relaxation training and guided imagery in reducing chemotherapy side effects in patients with breast cancer and in improving their quality of life. Support Care Cancer 2005;13(10): 826–33.

[69] Bakke AC, Purtzer MZ, Newton P. The effect of hypnotic-guided imagery on psychological well-being and immune function in patients with prior breast cancer. J Psychosom Res. 2002;53:1131–7.

[70] Leon-Pizzara C, Gich I, Barthe E, et al. A randomized trial of the effect of training in relaxation and guided imagery techniques in improving psychological and quality-of-life indices for gynecologic and breast brachytherapy patients. Psychooncology 2007;16(11): 971–9.

[71] Newton BW. The use of hypnosis in the treatment of cancer patients. Am J Clin Hypn 1982–1983;25(2–3):105–9.

[72] Spiegel D, Moore R. Imagery and hypnosis in the treatment of cancer patients. Oncol 1997;11(8):1179–89.

[73] Spiegel D. The use of hypnosis in controlling cancer pain. CA Cancer J Clin 1985;35(4): 221–31.

[74] Marcus J, Elkins G, Mott M. A model of hypnotic intervention for palliative care. Adv Mind Body Med 2003;19(2):24–7.

[75] Rheingans J. A systematic review of nonpharmacologic adjunctive therapies for symptom management in children with cancer. J Pediatr Oncol Nurs 2007;24:81–94.

[76] Feldman CS, Salzberg HC. The role of imagery in the hypnotic treatment of adverse reactions to cancer therapy. J S C Med Assoc 1990 May;86(5):303–6.

[77] Richardson J, Smith JE, McCall G, et al. Hypnosis for nausea and vomiting in cancer chemotherapy; a systematic review of the research evidence. Eur J Cancer Care (Engl) 2007;16(5):402–12.

[78] Marchioro G, Azzarello G, Viviani F, et al. Hypnosis in the treatment of anticipatory nausea and vomiting in patients receiving cancer chemotherapy. Oncol 2C ⁓⁓·⁻ ⁻:100–4.

[79] Taylor E, Ingleton C. Hypnotherapy and cognitive behaviour therapy in cancer care: the patients' view. Eur J Cancer Care (Engl) 2003;12:137–42.

[80] Montgomery GH, Bovbjerg DH, Schnur JB, et al. A randomized clinical trial of a brief hypnosis intervention to control side effects in breast surgery patients. J Natl Cancer Inst 2007;99(17):1304–12.

[81] Miller N. The dumb autonomic nervous system, and biofeedback. In: Dienstfrey H, editor. Where the mind meets the body. New York: HarperCollins; 1991.

[82] Basmajian JV, editor. Biofeedback: principles and practice for clinicians. 3rd editon. Baltimore: Williams and Wilkins; 1989.

[83] Hatch JP, Fisher JG, Rugh JD. Biofeedback: studies in clinical efficacy. New York: Plenum; 1987.

[84] Burgio KL, Goode PS, Urban DA, et al. Preoperative biofeedback assisted behavioral training to decrease post-prostatectomy incontinence: a randomized, controlled trial. J Urol 2006;175(1):196–201.

[85] NIH technology assessment panel on integration of behavioral and relaxation approaches into the treatment of chronic pain and insomnia. JAMA 1996;276:313–8.

[86] Tsai PS, Chen PL, Lai YL, et al. Effects of electromyography biofeedback-assisted relaxation on pain in patients with advanced cancer in a palliative care unit. Cancer Nurs 2007;30(5):347–53.

[87] Burcish TG. Effectiveness of biofeedback and relaxation training in reducing the side effects of cancer chemotherapy. Health Psychol 1992;11:17–23.

[88] Norris PA, Fahrion SL. Autogenic biofeedback in psychophysiological therapy and stress management. In: Leher PM, Woodfolk RL, editors. Principles and practices of stress management. New York: The Guildford Press; 1993. p. 231–62.

[89] Hidderley M, Holt M. A pilot randomized trial assessing the effects of autogenic training in early stage cancer patients in relation to psychological status and immune system responses. Eur J Oncol Nurs 2004;8:61–5.

[90] Stetter F, Kupper S. Autogenic training: a meta-analysis of clinical studies. Appl Psychophysiol Biofeedback 2002;27(1):45–98.

[91] Stanton AL, Danoff-Burg S, Sworowski LA, et al. Randomized controlled trial of written emotional expression and benefit finding in breast cancer patients. J Clin Oncol 2002;20(20): 4160–8.

[92] Pennebaker JW, Colder M, Sharp LK. Accelerating the coping process. J Pers Soc Psychol. 1990;58(3):528–37.

[93] Pennebaker JW. Putting stress into words: health, linguistic, and therapeutic implications. Behav Res Ther 1993;31(6):539–48.

[94] Pennebaker JW, Kiecolt-Glaser JK, Glaser R. Disclosure of traumas and immune function: health implications for psychotherapy. J Pers Soc Psychol 1988;63:75–84.

[95] Smyth JM, Stone AA, Hurewitz A, Kaell A. Effects of writing about stressful experiences on symptom reduction in patients with asthma or rheumatoid arthritis. JAMA 1999;281(14): 1304–9.

[96] DeMoor C, Sterner J, Hall M, et al. A pilot study on the effects of expressive writing on psychological and behavioral adjustment in patients enrolled in a phase I trial of vaccine therapy for metastatic renal cell carcinoma. Health Psychol 2002;21(6):615–9.

[97] Rancour P, Brauer K. Use of letter writing as a means of integrating an altered body image: a case study. Oncol Nurs Forum 2003;30(5):841–6.

[98] Christie W, Moore C. The impact of humor on patients with cancer. Clin J Oncol Nurs 2004;9(2):211–8.

[99] Johnson P. The use of humor and its influences on spirituality and coping in breast cancer survivors. Oncol Nurs Forum 2002;29:691–5.

[100] Kash KM, Holland JC, Breitbart W, et al. Stress and burnout in oncology. Oncology 2000;14:1621–33.

[101] Rollins JA. Tell me about it: drawing as a communication tool for children with cancer. J Pediatr Oncol Nurs 2005;22:203–21.

[102] Horstman M, Bradding A. Helping children speak up in the health service. Eur J Oncol Nurs 2002;6(2):75–84.

[103] Favara-Scacco C, Smirne G, Schilirò G, Di Cataldo A. Art therapy as support for children with leukemia during painful procedures. Med Pediatr Oncol 2000;36:474–80.

[104] Borgmann E. Art therapy with three women diagnosed with cancer. Arts in Psychotherapy 2002;29(5):245–51.

[105] Nainis N, Paice JA, Ratner J, et al. Relieving symptoms in cancer: innovative use of art therapy. J Pain Symptom Manage 2006;31(2):162–8.

[106] Oster I, Svensk AC, Magnusson E, et al. Art therapy improves coping resources: a randomized, controlled study among women with breast cancer. Palliat Support Care 2006;4: 57–64.

[107] Knols R, Aaronson N, Uebelhart D. Physical exercise in cancer patients during and after medical treatment: a systematic review of randomized and controlled clinical trials. J Clin Oncol 2005;23(16):3830–42.

[108] McNeely ML, Campbell KL, Rowe BH. Effects of exercise on breast cancer patients and survivors: a systematic review and meta-analysis. CMAJ 2006;175(1):34–41.

[109] Courneya KS, Mackey JR, Bell GJ, et al. Randomized controlled trial of exercise training in postmenopausal breast cancer survivors: cardiopulmonary and quality of life outcomes. J Clin Oncol 2003;21:1660–8.

[110] Courneya KS, Keats MR, Turner AR. Physical exercise and quality of life in cancer patients following high dose chemotherapy and autologous bone marrow transplantation. Psychooncology 2000;9(2):127–36.

[111] Courneya KS, Friedenreich CM. Physical exercise and quality of life following cancer diagnosis: a literature review. Ann Behav Med 1999;21(2):171–9.

[112] Turner JT, Hayes S, Reul-Hirche H. Improving the physical status and quality of life of women treated for breast cancer: a pilot study of a structured exercise intervention. J Surg Oncol 2004;86:141–6.

[113] Demark-Wahnefried W, Clipp EC, Morey MC, et al. Physical function and associations with diet and exercise: results of a cross-sectional survey among elders with breast cancer or prostate cancer. Int J Behav Nutr Phys Act 2004;29;1(1):16.

[114] Adamsen L, Midtgaard J, Andersen C, et al. Transforming the nature of fatigue through exercise: qualitative findings from a multidimensional exercise programme in cancer patients undergoing chemotherapy. Eur J Cancer Care 2004;13:362–70.

[115] Oldervoll LM, Kaasa S, Knobel H, Loge JH. Exercise reduces fatigue in chronic fatigued Hodgkins disease survivors-results from a pilot study. Eur J Cancer 2002;39:57–63.

[116] Blanchard CM, Baker F, Denniston MM, et al. Is absolute amount or change in exercise more associated with quality of life in adult cancer survivors. Prev Med 2003;37(5):389–96.

[117] Courneya KS, Friedenreich CM, Sela RA, Quinney HA, Rhodes RE, Handman M. The group psychotherapy and home-based physical exercise (group-hope) trial in cancer survivors: physical fitness and quality of life outcomes. Psychooncology 2003;12(4): 357–74.

[118] Courneya KS. A randomized trial of exercise and quality of life in colorectal cancer survivors. Eur J Cancer Care (Engl) 2003;12:347–57.

[119] Courneya KS. Exercise in cancer survivors: an overview of research. Med Sci Sports Exerc 2003;35(11):1846–52.

[120] LaFontaine TP, DiLorenzo TM, Frensch PA, et al. Aerobic exercise and mood. A brief review. Sports Med 1992;13(3):160–70.

[121] Mock V, Dow KH, Meares CJ, et al. Effects of exercise on fatigue, physical functioning, and emotional distress during radiation therapy for breast cancer. Oncol Nurs Forum 1997;24(6):991–1000.

[122] Matthews CE, Shu XO, Jin F, et al. Lifetime physical activity and breast cancer risk in the Shanghai Breast Cancer Study. Br J Cancer 2001;84(7):994–1001.

[123] McTiernan A, Kooperberg C, White E, et al. Recreational physical activity and the risk of breast cancer in postmenopausal women: The Women's Health Initiative Cohort Study. JAMA 2003;290:1331–5.

[124] Nilsen TI, Vatten LJ. Prospective study of colorectal cancer risk and physical activity, diabetes, blood glucose and BMI: exploring the hyperinsulinaemia hypothesis. Br J Cancer 2001;84(3):417–22.

[125] Rockhill B, Willett WC, Hunter DJ, et al. A prospective study of recreational physical activity and breast cancer risk. Arch Intern Med 1999;159(19):2290–6.

[126] Tavani A, Gallus S, La Vecchia C, et al. Physical activity and risk of ovarian cancer: an Italian case-control study. Int J Cancer 2001;91(3):407–11.

[127] Thune I, Lund E. Physical activity and risk of colorectal cancer in men and women. Br J Cancer 1996;73(9):1134–40.

[128] Bower JE, Woolery A, Sternlieb B, et al. Yoga for cancer patients and survivors. Cancer Control 2005;12:165–71.

[129] Culos-Reed SN, Carlson LE, Daroux LM, et al. A pilot study of yoga for breast cancer survivors: physical and psychological benefits. Psychooncology 2006;15:891–7.

[130] Cohen L, Warneke C, Fouladi R, et al. Psychological adjustment and sleep quality in a randomized trial of the effects of a Tibetan yoga intervention in patients with lymphoma. Cancer 2004;100:2253–60.

[131] Gopinath KS, Rao R, Raghuram N, et al. Evaluation of yoga therapy as a psychotherapeutic intervention in breast cancer patients on conventional combined modality of treatment. Proceedings of the 39th Annual Meeting of the American Society of Clinical Oncology (ASCO); 2003 May 31–Jun 3; Chicago, IL. p. 26.

[132] Carson JW, Carson KM, Porter LS, et al. Yoga for women with metastatic breast cancer: results from a pilot study. J Pain Symptom Manage 2007;33(3):331–41.

[133] Moadel AB, Shah C, Wylie-Roett J, et al. Randomized controlled trial of yoga among multiethnic sample of breast cancer patients: effects on quality of life. J Clin Oncol 2007;25(28):4387–95.

[134] Berkman LF, Syme SL. Social networks, host resistance and mortality: a nine-year follow-up study of Alameda county residents. Am J Epidemiol 1979;109(2):186–204.

[135] Kiecolt-Glaser JK, Glaser R. Stress and immune function in humans. In: Ader R, Felten D, Cohen N, editors. Psychoneuroimmunology II. San Diego: Academic Press; 1991. p. 849–67.

[136] Kiecolt-Glaser JK, Cacioppo JT, Malarkey WB, et al. Acute psychological stressors and short-term immune changes: what, why, for whom, and to what extent? Psychosom Med 1992;54:680–5.

[137] Maunsell E, Brisson J, Deschênes L. Social support and survival among women with breast cancer. Cancer 1995;76:631–7.

[138] Brown-Saltzman K. Replenishing the spirit by meditative prayer and guided imagery. Semin Oncol Nurs 1997;13(4):255–9.

[139] Investigating the epidemiologic effects of religious experience: findings, explanations, and barriers. In: Levin JS, editor. Religion in aging and health: theoretical foundations and methodological frontiers. Thousand Oaks (CA): A Sage Publications; 1994. p. 3–17.

[140] Levin JS. Religious factors in aging, adjustment and health: a theoretical overview. In: Clements WM, editor. Religion, aging, and health: a global perspective. New York: Haworth; 1989. p. 83–103.

[141] Levin JS, Vanderpool HY. Religious factors in physical health and the prevention of illness. In: Pargament KI, Maton KI, Hess RE, editors. Religion and prevention in mental health: research, vision, and action. New York: Haworth; 1992. p. 83–103.

[142] Spiegel D, Bloom JR, Yalom I. Group support for patients with metastatic cancer. Arch Gen Psychiatry 1981;38:527–33.

[143] Spiegel D, Bloom JR, Kraemer HC, Gottheil E. Effect of psychosocial treatment on survival of patients with metastatic breast cancer. Lancet 1989;2:888–91.

[144] Fawzy F, Fawzy NW, Hyun CS, et al. Malignant melanoma: effects of an early structured psychiatric intervention, coping, and affective state on recurrence and survival 6 years later. Arch Gen Psychiatry 1993;50:681–9.

[145] Fawzy F, Cousins N, Fawzy NW, Kemeny ME, Elashoff R, Morton D. A structured psychiatric intervention for cancer patients: I. Changes over time in methods of coping and affective disturbance. Arch Gen Psychiatry 1990;47:720–5.

[146] Fawzy F, Kemeny ME, Fawzy NW, et al. A structured psychiatric intervention for cancer patients: II. Changes over time in immunological measures. Arch Gen Psychiatry 1990;47:729–35.

[147] Richardson JL, Shelton DR, Krailo M, Levine AM. The effect of compliance with treatment on survival among patients with hematologic malignancies. J Clin Oncol 1990;14(4): 1128–35.

[148] Goodwin PJ, Leszcz M, Ennis M, et al. The effect of group psychological support on survival in metastatic breast cancer. N Engl J Med 2001;34:1719–26.

[149] Spiegel D, Butler LD, Giese-Davis J, et al. Effects of supportive-expressive group therapy on survival of patients with metastatic breast cancer: a randomized prospective trial. Cancer 2007;110(5):1130–8.

[150] Cunningham AJ. How psychological therapy may prolong survival in cancer patients. Integr Cancer Ther 2004;3(3):214–29.

[151] Cunningham AJ, Phillips C, Lockwood GA, et al. Association of involvement in psychological self-regulation with longer survival in patients with metastatic cancer: an exploratory study. Adv Mind Body Med 2000;16(4):276–87.

[152] Cunningham AJ, Edmonds CV, Phillips C, et al. A prospective, longitudinal study of the relationship of psychological work to duration of survival in patients with metastatic cancer. Psychooncology 2000;9(4):323–39.

Hematol Oncol Clin N Am 22 (2008) 709–725

Practical Hypnotic Interventions During Invasive Cancer Diagnosis and Treatment

Nicole Flory, PhD*,1, Elvira Lang, MD, FSIR, FSCEH

Department of Radiology, Beth Israel Deaconess Medical Center, Harvard Medical School, One Deaconess Road, Boston, MA 02215, USA

Over the past decade, numerous advances have been made in the diagnosis and treatment of cancer. A revolution in medical imaging and biomedical technology has enabled earlier detection, more targeted therapy, and the replacement of traditional large incision surgery with "minimally invasive" procedures. Interventional radiologists, surgeons, gastroenterologists, urologists, and pulmonologists (to name the representatives of just a few of the specialties involved) use these types of procedures to access tumor tissue. Due to the delicate nature of the intervention, all of these specialties require patients to be cooperative and to hold still, sometimes for hours. "Moderate" or "conscious" sedation with analgesics and sedatives has replaced the need for general anesthesia in common practice [1], allowing the patient to be an awake participant attended by the procedure team.

Although considered technically minimally invasive, these procedures still involve psychologic and physical strain on patients. Patients may experience anticipatory anxiety about being in pain, losing control, reacting to anesthesia, the destruction of body image, the disruption of life plans, and death [2]. Friends and relatives may also have difficulties adapting, which may leave patients to cope on their own [3]. In the hectic modern medical environment, the procedure room may be the only place where a patient can voice concerns in a confidential environment [4]. Having the procedure team prepared to provide effective support in a timely manner is an opportunity that should not be missed. Based on the authors' experience, procedural hypnosis can be an effective tool for reducing pain, anxiety, medication side effects, and complications.

This work was supported by the National Institutes of Health (RO1 AT-0002-05), the National Center for Complementary and Alternative Medicine (K24 AT01074-01), and the Ruth L. Kirschstein National Research Service Award, National Institutes of Health and National Institute of Cancer (T32-59367).

1Address after October 15, 2008: 16 Gardner St., Arlington, MA 02474.

*Corresponding author. E-mail address: nflory@bidmc.harvard.edu (N. Flory).

0889-8588/08/$ – see front matter
doi:10.1016/j.hoc.2008.04.008

ANTICIPATORY EMOTIONS

Anxiety about upcoming medical interventions can be distressing. Even patients waiting to undergo a "simple" diagnostic procedure such as image-guided breast biopsy have greatly elevated anxiety levels [5–7]. Facing breast cancer may be particularly distressing because of the potential for loss of body image [2] and the high frequency rate (31%) of all cancers in women [8], which increases the likelihood of knowing a breast cancer patient or survivor. In fact, data from 253 women awaiting radiology procedures show that women awaiting breast biopsy report significant more anxiety than women before embolization of benign uterine fibroids or malignancies of the liver (Nicole Flory, S. Faintuch, E.V. Lang, unpublished data, 2008). Women awaiting breast biopsy also report heightened depressive symptoms and general psychologic distress compared with normative data from nonclinical samples (Nicole Flory, S. Faintuch, E.V. Lang, unpublished data, 2008). Depressive mood and perceived stress ratings in biopsy patients were comparable to women who had diagnosed cancers of the liver undergoing chemoembolization and significantly elevated compared with uterine fibroid embolization.

Hospitals providing high-tech procedures such as CT scans for cancer patients would best be advised to include psychologic support and enhanced communication with patients because the complexity of radiologic procedures has grown [9]. The anticipatory anxiety of patients not only magnifies patients' intraprocedural anxiety but also affects patients' pain during the procedure [10]. Furthermore, anticipatory anxiety is a predictor of medication use during the procedure. Individuals who are very anxious and distressed at the outset tend to receive more medication with or without requesting it [10], which may result in oversedation of patients that may become evident only after the procedure when the intraoperative emotional arousal no longer masks the drug effects [11]. Patients who have higher initial anxiety may therefore be more prone to adverse drug effects and related symptoms.

Pain and distress may lead not only to the additional use of medication but also to longer hospital stays and readmissions [12]. Schupp and colleagues [10] demonstrated a significant positive correlation between anticipatory anxiety and procedure length. An unsuccessful recovery from surgery not only adversely affects patient but also inflates health care costs [13]. It is unfortunate that patients' perceptions may sometimes become self-fulfilling prophecies. Benotsch [14] assessed personality characteristics that could adversely affect patients' experience during invasive procedures and found that negative affect was the most powerful predicator of procedural pain, anxiety, drug use, and complications.

POWER OF SUGGESTION

When receiving medical care, patients are not only often anxious but also highly suggestible [15]. In this setting, they may become particularly attuned to the verbal and nonverbal cues in their environment [16]. The fears of the cancer patients and those of their family, friends, and helpers regarding possible complications and death should not be underestimated, and communication may become strained [3]. When reviewing tapes of interventional radiology procedures, it is evident that patients are distressed and that personnel often seem tense and attempt to lighten the atmosphere by gentle jokes or nervous laughter [17].

Health care providers in cancer care are advised to pay attention to what their words may be suggesting to patients, whether or not a formal hypnotic induction is used [15]. Negative suggestions include many statements commonly used in the daily routine of the hospital, such as "little sting here" or "sharp scratch there" [4]. Lang and colleagues [18] videotaped 159 interventional radiology procedures and analyzed the interactions between patients and health care providers. Warning the patient about upcoming stimuli and potentially painful and unpleasant experiences resulted in significantly greater pain and anxiety than not doing so. Negatively loaded statements can become self-fulfilling prophecies that create the very same adverse outcomes health professionals try to avoid [18]. Herbert Spiegel [15] described the most striking example of this in the premature death of a patient who had been mistaken by the priest for his hospital roommate and who erroneously received the last rites. Such outcomes have been described as the "nocebo" effect [15]. Statements like "now, we are putting you to sleep" can recall unwanted associations in a pediatric cancer patient about her dog that was "put asleep" by the veterinarian. Therefore, emotionally positive or neutral descriptions are preferable to negative suggestions. Neutral descriptors include "some feeling of warmth, coolness, or tingling" [5]. Positive suggestions such as "would you like to go into relaxation more quickly or slowly" foster the patient's well-being during the procedures [18]. Immunizing comments such as "use only the suggestions that are helpful to you" can prevent harm from negative suggestions [4].

Knowing how to improve patients' comfort during invasive procedures not only increases the subjective well-being of patients but also facilitates the technical aspects of the procedure. Patients' anxiety can be reduced through psychologic and pharmacologic interventions [11]. Pharmacologic agents such as sedatives, narcotics, and analgesics are typically quick to apply and fast acting [1]. These agents, however, can also cause serious side effects and require cautious monitoring, particularly in pediatric patients [19]. Nonpharmacolgic interventions such as brief cognitive behavioral or hypnotic techniques are safe and carry little risk for adverse effects [20].

RESEARCH EVIDENCE

Patients often go through different phases of cancer-related issues, including initial symptoms, diagnostic testing, diagnosis, various acute and longer-term treatment modalities, and coping with longer-term consequences and sometimes palliative care. During the various stages of diagnosis and treatment, different aspects are at the forefront of concern for cancer patients and their helpers. These concerns may range from anticipatory anxiety, procedural anxiety, acute and chronic pain, procedural complications, nausea, emesis, and others [21]. Pharmacologic and nonpharmacologic treatments have their place in battling these symptoms.

In the procedure room, the needs of the patient and the intervention team intersect, with each bringing their own perspectives, hopes, and experiences to the operating table. In addition to psychologic comfort, safety becomes paramount. It is no simple task for the patient to remain immobilized, calm, and cooperative while being operated on in the midst of strangers in a cold procedure room full of high-tech instruments and equipment. Particularly when technical challenges or complications deviate from planned intervention, the ability of the patient and team to remain calm and resourceful can greatly affect outcome. The authors, therefore, look at the evidence in terms of patient comfort, safety, and behavior in relation to the behavior of the treatment team [17,18].

In recent years, the usefulness of hypnotic techniques in conjunction with pharmacologic treatments during invasive surgery has been investigated [22]. The effectiveness of hypnotic interventions has been documented in different phases of treatment: during diagnostic large-core breast biopsy [5], before breast biopsy or lumpectomy [13], during invasive interventional radiologic procedures [23], during percutaneous tumor treatments such as tumor embolizations and radiofrequency ablations [17], and after ambulatory surgery in children [24]. Based on a meta-analysis of hypnosis for surgery, Montgomery and colleagues [22] concluded that on average, 89% of patients profited from adjunctive hypnosis compared with standard care. The beneficial effects of hypnosis were documented in all investigated areas of patient welfare: pain, pain medication, physiologic indicators, recovery, treatment time, and emotional well-being. Faymonville and colleagues [25] documented similar benefits of adjunctive hypnosis in their analysis of retrospective and prospective studies in which they reviewed 1650 cases of patients undergoing different medical procedures. Recent reviews of the literature suggest that adults and children can greatly benefit from hypnosis during cancer treatment, although there is a need for further research on the effectiveness of hypnosis for procedural pain and distress in pediatric oncology patients [26,27].

Several prospective randomized controlled trials (RCTs) with samples of 200 or more patients undergoing invasive treatments have now been published (Table 1). Lang and colleagues [5] conducted a prospective RCT on hypnosis for 236 women undergoing diagnostic testing for breast cancer (large-core breast biopsy). Patients were randomized to receive (in addition to local anesthetic and while on the procedure table) standard care, empathic attention, or self-hypnotic relaxation treatment. In the two latter conditions, an additional team member stayed with the patient throughout the procedure displaying structured empathic attention behaviors or, in the hypnosis condition, reading a hypnosis script. This script was originally developed by David Spiegel and was used with modifications in three prospective RCTs [5,17,23]. It uses an eye roll induction in which the patient is invited to roll up the eyes, close the eyes, and focus on a sensation of floating. The patient is then instructed to experience with all senses his or her chosen imagery. If needed, provisions

| Table 1 | | | | | | |
| Hypnosis for pain and anxiety during medical procedures | | | | | | |
Study	N	Design	Procedure	Control treatment	Results	Additional information
Lang et al [23]	241	RCT	Renal and vascular radiology interventions in adults	Empathic attention Standard care	Significant; hypnosis resulted in reduced P/A, medication use, and procedure time compared with standard care	Largest N; hypnosis significantly reduced costs ($330 savings per patient compared with standard care); hypnosis also resulted in a significantly greater hemodynamic stability
Lang et al [5]	236	RCT	Breast biopsy in adults	Empathic attention Standard care	Significant; hypnosis resulted in reduced P/A compared with standard care; empathic attention resulted in reduced pain only	Room time and costs were not significantly different between groups even though hypnosis and empathy groups required an additional professional
Montgomery et al [13]	200	RCT	Breast surgery in adults	Attention control	Significant; hypnosis resulted in reduced pain, fatigue, discomfort, and "emotional upset"	Hypnosis significantly reduced costs for the institution, mostly due to reduced surgery time ($772 savings per patient compared with control)
Lang et al [17]	201	RCT	Percutaneous tumor treatment in adults	Empathic attention Standard care	Significant; hypnosis resulted in reduced, P/A, and medication use compared with standard care and empathic attention	Empathic attention was associated with significantly more adverse events compared with hypnosis and standard care

Results based on prospective RCTs with N≥200.
Abbreviation: P/A, pain and anxiety.

Box 1: Hypnosis study script

The following provides illustrations for the use of hypnotic techniques during
  medical procedures. Only health care professionals who have received
  comprehensive training in hypnosis should use these techniques.

Brief explanation

"We want you to help us to help you learn a concentration exercise to help you
  get through the procedure more comfortably. It is just a form of concentration,
  like getting so caught up in a movie or a good book that you forget you are
  watching a movie or reading a book."

Immunization against noise and negative suggestions

"If you hear sounds or noises in the room, just use these exercises to deepen your
  experience and use only the suggestions that are helpful to you."

Brief induction

"There are a lot of ways to relax but here is one simple way: On one, you can do
  one thing—look up. On two, two things—slowly close your eyes and take
  a deep breath. On three, three things—breath out, relax your eyes, and let
  your body float. That's good. Just imagine your whole body floating, floating
  through the table, each breath deeper and easier."

Develop positive imagery

"Right now you might imagine that you are floating somewhere safe and comfortable, in a bath, a lake, a hot tub, or just floating in space, each breath deeper
  and easier. Just notice how with each breath you let a little more tension out of
  your body as you let your whole body float, safe and comfortable, each breath
  deeper and easier. Good. Now, with your eyes closed and remaining in this
  state of concentration, please describe for me how your body is feeling right
  now. Where do you imagine yourself being; what is it like? Can you smell
  the air? Can you see what is around you?"

Anchoring in resourceful imagery

"Good. Now, this is your safe and pleasant place to be and you can use it in
  a sense to play a trick on the doctors. Your body has to be here, but you
  don't. So, just spend your time being somewhere you would rather be."

Immunization against discomfort

"Now, if there is some discomfort, and there may be some with the procedure,
  there is no point in fighting it. You can admit it, but then transform that sensation. If you feel some discomfort, you might find it helpful to make that part
  of your body to feel warmer, as if you were in a bath. Or cooler, if that is
  more comfortable, as if you had ice or snow on that part of your body. Or
  you may experience a tingling sensation on that body part. This warmth, coolness, or tingling sensation becomes a protective filter between you and the
  discomfort."

Check in with patient

"Now, again with your eyes closed and remaining in the state of concentration,
  describe what your are feeling right now."

If they are at their safe and comfortable place, reinforce it: "What is it like now? What do you see around you? What are you doing?"

If they are in pain: "The pain is there but see if you can add coolness, more warmth, or make it lighter or heavier."

If not in pain: "Good. Continue to focus on these sensations."

If still in pain: "Now, imagine yourself being at _____ (use resourceful positive imagery) where you said you felt relaxed and comfortable. What is it like now? What is the temperature? What do you see around you?"

If they state that they are worried: "Okay, your main job right now is to help your body feel comfortable, so we will talk about what is worrying you. But first, no matter what we discuss, concentrate on your body floating. So, let's get the floating back into your body. Imagine that you are in this favorite spot and when you are ready, let me know by nodding your head and then we will talk about what is worrying you. But remember no matter what we discuss, concentrate on your body floating, and feel safe and comfortable. So what is worrying you? (Discuss).

Check in with patient

"How do you feel now?"

If comfortable: "Good. Now, continue to concentrate on body floating, and feel safe and comfortable in your favorite place."

If uncomfortable, use the split-screen technique: "Okay, you might picture in your mind a screen like a movie screen, TV screen, or a piece of clear blue sky. First, you might see a pleasant scene on it. Now you may picture a large piece of blue screen divided in half. All right, on the left half, picture what you are worrying about on the screen. On the right half, picture what you will do about it, or what you would recommend someone else to do about it. Keep your body floating, and if you are worrying about the outcome, it is okay to admit it to yourself, but your body does not have to get uptight about it. You may, but your body does not have to. Good. You know that whatever happens, there is always something you can do. But for now, just concentrate on keeping your body floating and feeling safe and comfortable."

Reorientation of patient

"The procedure is over now. We are going to formally leave this state of concentration by counting backward from three to one. On three, get ready; on two with your eyes closed, roll up your eyes; and on one, let your eyes open and take a deep breath and let it out. That will be the end of the formal exercise, but when you come out of it you will still have the feeling of comfort that you felt during it. Ready: three, two, one."

to dispel any anxiety or pain are included. Box 1 outlines the hypnosis induction script and Fig. 1 provides an algorithm outlining the operationalization of hypnosis on the procedure table. With the use of this script, Lang and colleagues [5] found that hypnosis during breast biopsy significantly reduced a patient's pain and anxiety, whereas empathic attention resulted in a reduction of pain ratings only. Findings from this study overlap with results from the most

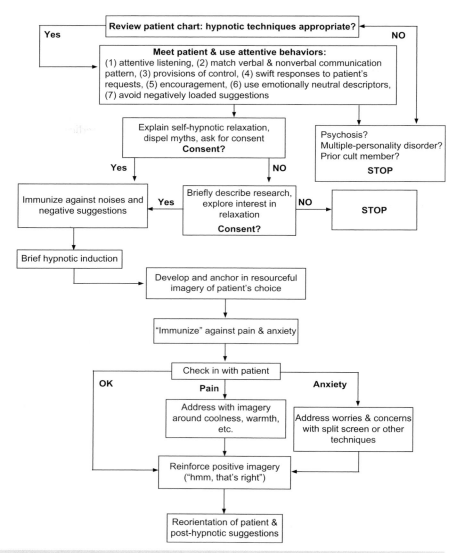

Fig. 1. An algorithm for the use of hypnotic techniques during an invasive procedure.

comprehensive RCT to date, which included 241 patients undergoing invasive procedures in interventional radiology [23]. Patients underwent interventions in the vasculature and the kidneys for benign and malignant conditions; they received standard care, empathic attention, or self-hypnotic relaxation using the same type of hypnosis script. Hypnosis significantly reduced pain, anxiety, and the use of pharmacologic agents. In addition, the rate of complications decreased, and time in the procedure room was reduced by 17 minutes in the hypnotic condition. According to a cost analysis for this RCT by Lang and Rosen [28], the average cost for procedures using adjunct hypnosis was $300, whereas the cost for procedures in the standard care group averaged $638. This difference resulted in significant cost savings for the procedures conducted under hypnosis, even when taking into account additional costs for a hypnosis provider [28]. In the most recent RCT comparing hypnosis, empathic attention, and standard care during percutaneous tumor treatment, Lang and colleagues [17] found that hypnosis reduced pain, anxiety, and medication use in this more invasive and challenging setting.

Montgomery and colleagues [13] conducted an RCT on 200 women undergoing lumpectomy of the breast. The investigators randomized patients to receive standard care, attention control, or hypnosis before entering the operating room. Hypnosis was provided by a psychologist in a 15-minute session. Hypnosis resulted in much more favorable outcomes for pain, fatigue, nausea, procedural discomfort, and emotional well-being than the other conditions. In addition, patients in the hypnosis group also requested and received less medication for sedation or pain. Time in the procedure room was also significantly reduced in the hypnosis condition. All of these favorable outcomes not only benefited the patient but also saved the hospital $770 per procedure [13]. These findings replicate similar results from an earlier RCT with 20 women undergoing excisional breast biopsy in which hypnosis reduced postoperative pain and distress [29].

Although several larger RCTs have demonstrated the effectiveness of hypnotic techniques to reduce pain and anxiety as stated previously and as shown in Table 1, findings with regard to nausea and emesis have yielded mixed results (Table 2). Several studies showed that hypnosis did not have much of an impact [30–32], but other studies demonstrated significant benefits with regard to emesis and nausea [13,33,34]. Pinnell and Covino's [35] review of the literature from 2000 indicated that hypnosis could be useful for reducing nausea and emesis; however, research findings were scarce and inconsistent then. A more recent review by Neron and Stephenson [21] from 2007 also stated that the literature on hypnosis for nausea and emesis is still too sparse and has too few patient numbers to draw final conclusions. Because cancer treatments have become more aggressive in the past 20 years, patients are in need of support (in particular, nonpharmacologic behavioral interventions) to manage associated symptoms [36]. Nausea and emesis are common during and after invasive procedures, and further attention to their management is warranted [37]. A recent prospective randomized trial by Montgomery and colleagues [13] of 200 women having lumpectomy or biopsy for breast cancer management was able to shed light on procedural nausea. There was a significant reduction in nausea for patients in the hypnosis group versus the control group (mean 6.7 versus 25.5 reported on visual analog scales from 0–100) [13].

INVOLVING THE WHOLE TREATMENT TEAM

Despite the scientific evidence from multiple RCTs, the acceptance of hypnotic techniques in operative cancer care has been slow. Considering that the

Table 2
Hypnosis for nausea and emesis during medical procedures

Authors	N	Design	Procedure	Control treatment	Results	Additional information
Zeltzer et al [34]	54	RCT	Chemotherapy in children	Cognitive distraction Therapist attention	Significant; hypnosis resulted in the greatest reduction in anticipatory and postchemotherapy symptoms, including N/E	Cognitive distraction group had nonhypnotic relaxation; attention control group had casual conversation with therapist
Syrjala et al [30]	67	RCT	Bone marrow transplant in adults	Cognitive-behavioral intervention Therapist contact Standard care	No significant difference for N/E, with no difference between groups, but hypnosis significantly reduced pain	Only 45 patients completed study; very small N in each group [10–12]; underpowered?
Ghoneim et al [31]	60	RCT	Molar surgery/ adults	Standard care	No significant difference for emesis, with no difference between groups, but hypnosis significantly reduced anxiety	Hypnosis was delivered by way of audiotape recordings; life hypnosis provider more effective?
Oddby-Muhrbeck et al [32]	70	RCT	Elective breast surgery in adults	Patients listened to a "blank" tape with low background music	No significant difference between groups in a 24-h period, but hypnosis group significantly less often recalled N/E	Hypnosis was delivered by way of tape (affirmative suggestions with soft music); life hypnosis provider more effective?
Enqvist et al [33]	50	RCT	Elective breast surgery in adults	Standard care	Significant; hypnosis resulted in reduced N/E and analgesia use	Patients in hypnosis group listened to audiotape with higher frequency (4–6 times/d) than previous studies [31,32]
Montgomery et al [13]	200	RCT	Breast surgery	Attention control	Significant; hypnosis resulted in reduced nausea and other symptoms	Largest N; best study until now; hypnosis delivered in real time by "life" provider

Results based on prospective RCTs with N≥50.
Abbreviation: N/E, nausea and emesis.

effectiveness and the safety of periprocedural hypnosis have been shown in more than 1000 patients in cumulative large-scale prospective randomized trials, one may wonder why this is the case [5,13,17,22,23]. This slow acceptance is particularly surprising with regard to the proven usefulness of hypnosis for the management of acute and chronic pain [38]. David Spiegel [39] observed that if hypnosis were an analgesic or anxiolytic drug, the pharmaceutic industry would have advocated broad dissemination. Reluctance to integrate hypnosis into the tool kit may have several reasons [40]; for instance, negative associations with "brainwashing" or supernatural powers, reservations toward appearing "touchy feely" in the eyes of one's peers, reliance on technologic gadgets and drugs as quick fixes, and the need to address one's own fears surrounding illness and cancer. The successful implementation of hypnotic skills depends on the cooperation of everyone involved in the patient's care; in particular, those in a confined and high-pressure environment such as the interventional radiology suite. It takes "a whole village" to create change.

When introducing hypnosis in the procedure suite, the authors encountered what they early on would have labeled sabotage. Managing patients' pain and anxiety deeply touches a caregiver's belief systems and affects the core of caring. Typically, strong institutional philosophies determine such belief systems and actions [41]. For example, the amount of drugs that patients receive by nursing during invasive procedures is determined by institutional belief systems rather than by patient needs or physician guidance [41]. This practice is facilitated by the fact that hospital policies address issues of patient monitoring during sedation but do not prescribe dosages. One of the authors had the opportunity to witness how this dilemma played itself out after the merger of two hospitals. In one hospital, nursing heavily sedated patients and in the other, nursing preferred small dosages, with both groups staunchly defending their practice and accusing each other of poor patient care. This difference in drug administration applied only to dosages given before the patients experienced distress. After patients experienced pain, both groups became relatively reluctant to give higher dosages, reflecting findings of a prior study that showed that most drugs were given when patients' anxiety and pain scores were low [41] and that when patients voiced high pain and anxiety scores, they did not necessarily receive more drug delivery. Considering that it took over a year to reconcile the drug dosing habits of the two nursing teams after the merger, one may not be too surprised that the introduction of a mind-body technique may face even stiffer resistance.

Some members of the treatment team, especially when not trained in hypnosis and perhaps even suspicious of such practices, may attempt to be "extra nice" to the patient to show they care by chatting. The authors had to halt a recent prospective randomized hypnosis trial for percutaneous tumor treatment after enrolling 201 patients because of a high level of adverse events in the empathic attention control condition [17]. Of 65 patients in the empathy group, 31 (48%) had adverse events—significantly more than in the hypnosis (8/66 [12%]; $P = .0001$) and standard care groups (18/70 [26%]; $P = .0118$). It is of interest that hypnosis (which included empathic attention behavior) reduced pain, anxiety, and medication use; yet empathic approaches alone (which provided an external focus of attention) did not enhance patients' self-coping. When reviewing the videotaped session, it became clearer how empathic attention and hypnosis differed. In the empathy condition, nurses engaged to a greater extent in conversations with the patient and the empathic care provider. These frequent interactions were often of a conversational nature following patterns of social interactions. For example, when patients mentioned topics such as travel, careers, or health problems, nurses expressed understanding and sympathy by talking about their own experiences, travels, and on occasion, about terrible things that had happened to them or other people. Rather than being a pleasant distraction, such discussions may have evoked disinterest or outright distress. In the hypnosis group, the topics the patient mentioned were used to structure patient-desirable imagery. If these topics brought up distressing emotional content, underlying concerns were further explored by helping patients help themselves find solutions. The ability to do this would typically require extensive training in psychologic techniques. The researchers in the trial, however, were able to accomplish this with provisions in the hypnosis script, adherence to a treatment manual, and two 8-hour training sessions with subsequent supervised application. Hypnosis training may thus be the answer to improving communication in the procedure suite.

In further attempts to understand the empathy paradox in the tumor treatment trial, one also needs to reflect on the stressors that health care providers face vis-à-vis cancer and risks of invasive procedures [17]. Observing others in distress can produce an affective response, which is oriented to decrease distress of the observer and the suffering person. This reaction often elicits a behavioral response, which may be targeted toward providing comfort and reassurance or withdrawal [42]. The affective response to seeing others in pain can be documented on functional MRI, whereby the intensity of empathy positively correlates with activation of neural substrates [43]. This greater feeling for the patient, however, does not necessarily translate into better patient care [44]. Providing hypnosis in the procedure room may thus not only help the patient but also the entire team in managing their stress. Particularly during invasive cancer treatment, it was remarkable to see how quickly the entire atmosphere calmed after induction of hypnosis [17].

TRAINING HEALTH CARE PROFESSIONALS

To reduce resistance, facilitate communication, or decrease interpersonal conflicts, one may argue it would be best to deliver hypnosis through a member who is already part of the medical procedure team, as suggested by Blankfield [16]. Ideally, this individual would be familiar with the workings of the procedure room and have the opportunity to get acquainted with the patient before the procedure. It is unfortunate that the two goals of being familiar with the treatment team and with the patient are often mutually exclusive. As mentioned earlier, the interventional suite tends to be a busy environment in which one procedure is often followed by the next, giving personnel little time for activities outside of the procedure room. A psychologist or therapist working in a private practice setting has many more opportunities to get to know the patient but may have inaccurate perceptions of the proceedings in invasive cancer treatments and may not accompany the patient into the procedure suite. Training health care professionals across different disciplines in pharmacologic and nonpharmacologic interventions is ideal.

A major impediment to introduction of procedural hypnosis has been the traditional stance of the hypnosis societies that only physicians, psychologists, social workers, dentists, or nurses who have master's degrees should be trained. Members of the national hypnosis societies and their local subsidiaries such as the Society for Clinical and Experimental Hypnosis (SCEH) and the American Society of Clinical Hypnosis (ASCH) had forbidden their members to train medical technologists or nurses who have only a bachelor's degree; however, results from procedural hypnosis studies, the realization of the opportunity, and the activism of members have brought about the following changes: in 2006, the New England Society of Clinical Hypnosis changed its bylaws to enable training in procedural hypnosis and membership for licensed health care professionals who have a bachelor's degree, such as nurses, radiologic technologists, emergency medical technicians, or individuals with similar training. SCEH and ASCH are following this model and, it is hoped, will approve changes to their bylaws in 2008. These changes will greatly facilitate the ability to make procedural hypnosis available to larger patient numbers.

Although hypnotic techniques have a long-standing history of success in the operating room [25,45] and carry minimal risks for patients [20], recommendations for safety should be considered. Team members providing hypnotic interventions in the procedure room should carefully monitor the patient's response and minimize the potential for negative effects early; for example, by anchoring a patient in a safe scenario should an abreaction happen. As a general principle, health care providers should use hypnosis only as an adjunctive treatment for a service in which they are professionally trained in the first place (eg, cancer should never be treated solely through hypnotic techniques instead of conventional treatments). Hypnosis should also not be used as the final tool to manage psychologic distress or medical emergencies. Although psychotic patients typically are not very hypnotizable [46], it is advisable that only mental health professionals use hypnotic techniques with this population. Several authors have argued that successful training in hypnosis results in a smaller likelihood of adverse effects [20]; therefore, only health care professionals who have comprehensive training in procedural hypnosis should use these techniques.

HOW TO DO IT YOURSELF

Patients increasingly value complementary approaches as adjuncts to our technology-driven health care [47]. With evidence accumulating about the benefits of procedural hypnosis, what can a patient do to receive it? It would be beneficial for the cancer patient to find health care providers who are at least open to his or her wishes for a comprehensive treatment approach that integrates the physical and psychologic aspects of their care. Becoming informed about the research and clinical findings on procedural hypnosis would be helpful.

More "mind-body centers" are opening in prestigious institutions and savvy practices; it is advisable to seek out help from licensed health care professionals who have extensive training in hypnosis. When referring physicians and practices do not offer or are unaware of hypnosis practitioners, patients can consult the Web pages of the SCEH and the ASCH and their local affiliates. Hypnosis-trained psychologists and physicians can address cancer-related issues comprehensively and prepare individualized tapes in preparation for surgery. In the early diagnostic stages, before disease is confirmed, this approach is typically limited to patients who have extensive anxiety and distress, strong motivation, and financial means. After the cancer diagnosis, support groups that include expressive supportive therapy with hypnosis sessions can provide considerable help [48].

A variety of commercial books and tapes are now available to help patients prepare for surgery. By their nature, these contributions employ a "one size fits all" approach. Some succeed better in this than others by using permissive Ericksonian language that leaves the patients with their own options of interpretation rather than being authoritarian in suggestions that the patient may reject [49]. The tapes can be lengthy (80 minutes) [50] and often recommend multiple practice sessions that may be too time-consuming for some patients and boring after several repetitions. One product requires cooperation by the anesthesiologist and affirmation of positive outcome at the end of surgery, regardless of the success or complications following the intervention [51]. Larger studies on the use of such tapes are lacking; hypnotic interventions delivered in an interactive fashion by a "life" hypnosis provider may be more productive (see Table 2). One advantage of audiotapes, however, maybe that the patient is less exposed to negative suggestions and distraction from procedure personnel and can thus better focus on internal coping, which is associated with less sympathetic arousal and less risk of adverse empathy effects.

Using hypnosis as a sole means to effectively manage pain and other symptoms during open surgery is rare [52]; Wain [52] labeled such talented individuals as hypnosis virtuosos. Using self-hypnosis without any guidance by a hypnosis provider or a tape in the operating team is also a rarity but has been documented in a case study [53]. Such an approach usually is limited to patients who are already experienced with hypnosis. In this case, a hypnotic induction that is self-generated and easy to repeat (eg, the eye-roll or looking at spot on the wall) is helpful because disruptions during the procedure may arise. It has also been shown that patients under stress can enter trance spontaneously without formal induction [54]. In the do-it-yourself context, it is important to remain immune to well-meant interruptions by the treatment team. A preprocedure explanation and discussion with the surgical team is recommended.

SUMMARY

Hypnotic techniques not only combat psychologic symptoms such as procedural pain, anxiety, and distress but also reduce the need for sedation and pharmacologic regimens while stabilizing vital signs. All these benefits of hypnosis interventions come at no additional costs; growing evidence suggests cost savings when reductions in procedure length, room time, and medication use as a result of procedural hypnosis are taken into account. Implications of these findings involve recommendations for the patient's active participation during his or her cancer treatment and the training of health care professionals in mind-body therapies.

References

[1] Mueller PR, Wittenberg KH, Kaufman JA, et al. Patterns of anesthesia and nursing care for interventional radiology procedures: a national survey of physician practices and preferences. Radiology 1997;202:339–43.

[2] Anderson K, Masur F. Psychological preparation for invasive medical and dental procedures. J Behav Med 1983;6:1–40.

[3] Spiegel D. Living beyond limits. New York: Random House Publishing; 1995.

[4] Lang EV, Lutgendorf S, Logan H, et al. Nonpharmacologic analgesia and anxiolysis for interventional radiological procedures. Seminars in Interventional Radiology 1999;16: 113–23.

[5] Lang EV, Berbaum KS, Faintuch S, et al. Adjunctive self-hypnotic relaxation for outpatient medical procedures: a prospective randomized trial with women undergoing large core breast biopsy. Pain 2006;126:155–64.

[6] Maxwell JR, Bugbee ME, Wellisch D, et al. Imaging-guided core needle biopsy of the breast: study of psychological outcomes. Breast J 2000;6(1):53–61.

[7] Helbich TH, Dantendorfer K, Mostbeck GH, et al. Randomized comparison of sitting and prone positions for stereotactic fine-needle aspiration breast biopsy. Br J Surg 1996;83: 1252–5.

[8] Jemal A, Siegel R, Ward E, et al. Cancer statistics, 2006. CA Cancer J Clin 2006;56(2): 106–30.

[9] Peteet JR, Stomper PC, Murray-Ross D, et al. Emotional support for patients with cancer who are undergoing CT: semistructured interviews of patients at a cancer institute. Radiology 1992;182:99–102.

[10] Schupp C, Berbaum K, Berbaum M, et al. Pain and anxiety during interventional radiological procedures. Effect of patients' state of anxiety at baseline and modulation by nonpharmacologic analgesia adjuncts. J Vasc Interv Radiol 2005;16:1585–92.

[11] Hatsiopoulou O, Cohen RI, Lang EV. Postprocedure pain management of interventional radiology patients. J Vasc Interv Radiol 2003;14(11):1373–85.

[12] Chung F, Ritchie E, Su J. Postoperative pain in ambulatory surgery. Anesth Analg 1997;85(4):808–16.

[13] Montgomery GH, Bovbjerg DH, Schnur JB, et al. A randomized clinical trial of a brief hypnosis intervention to control side effects in breast surgery patients. J Natl Cancer Inst 2007;99(17):1304–12.

[14] Benotsch E. Individual differences and psychological preparation for invasive medical procedures. Thesis in Clinical Psychology. Iowa City (IA): The University of Iowa; 1998.

[15] Spiegel H. Nocebo: the power of suggestibility. Prev Med 1997;26:616–21.

[16] Blankfield RP. Suggestion, relaxation, and hypnosis as adjuncts in the care of surgery patients: a review of the literature. Am J Clin Hypn 1991;33:172–86.

[17] Lang EV, Berbaum KS, Pauker SG, et al. Beneficial effects of hypnosis and adverse effects of empathic attention during percutaneous tumor treatment. When being nice does not suffice. J Vasc Interv Radiol 2008;19(6):897–905.

[18] Lang EV, Hatsiopoulou O, Koch T, et al. Can words hurt? Patient-provider interactions during invasive procedures. Pain 2005;114(1–2):303–9.

[19] Yaster M, Cravero JP. The continuing conundrum of sedation for painful and nonpainful procedures. J Pediatr 2004;145:10–2.

[20] Lynn SJ, Martin DJ, Frauman DC. Does hypnosis pose special risks for negative effects? A master class commentary. Int J Clin Exp Hypn 1996;44:7–19.

[21] Neron S, Stephenson R. Effectiveness of hypnotherapy with cancer patients' trajectory: emesis, acute pain, and analgesia and anxiolysis in procedures. Int J Clin Exp Hypn 2007;55(3):336–54.

[22] Montgomery GH, David D, Winkel G, et al. The effectiveness of adjunctive hypnosis with surgical patients: a meta-analysis. Anesth Analg 2002;94:1639–45.

[23] Lang EV, Benotsch EG, Fick LJ, et al. Adjunctive non-pharmacologic analgesia for invasive medical procedures: a randomized trial. Lancet 2000;355:1486–90.

[24] Huth MM, Broome ME, Good M. Imagery reduces children's postoperative pain. Pain 2004;110:439–48.

[25] Faymonville ME, Meurisse M, Fissette J. Hypnosedation: a valuable alternative to traditional anaesthetic techniques. Acta Chir Belg 1999;99:141–6.

[26] Richardson J, Smith JE, McCall G, et al. Hypnosis for procedure-related pain and distress in pediatric cancer patients: a systematic review of effectiveness and methodology related to hypnosis interventions. J Pain Symptom Manage 2006;31(1):70–84.

[27] Wild MR, Espie CA. The efficacy of hypnosis in the reduction of procedural pain and distress in pediatric oncology: a systematic review. J Dev Behav Pediatr 2004;25(3):207–13.

[28] Lang EV, Rosen M. Cost analysis of adjunct hypnosis for sedation during outpatient interventional procedures. Radiology 2002;222:375–82.

[29] Montgomery GH, Weltz CR, Seltz M, et al. Brief presurgery hypnosis reduces stress and pain in excisional breast biopsy patients. Int J Clin Exp Hypn 2002;50:17–32.

[30] Syrjala KL, Cummings C, Donaldson GW, et al. Hypnosis or cognitive behavioral training for the reduction of pain and nausea during cancer treatment: a controlled clinical trial. Pain 1992;48:137–46.

[31] Ghoneim MM, Block RI, Sarasin DS, et al. Tape-recorded hypnosis instructions as adjuvant in the care of patients scheduled for third molar surgery. Anesth Analg 2000;90:64–8.

[32] Oddby-Muhrbeck E, Jakobsson J, Enquist B. Implicit processing and therapeutic suggestion during balanced anaesthesia. Acta Anaesthesiol Scand 1995;39(3):333–7.

[33] Enqvist B, Bjorklund C, Engman M, et al. Preoperative hypnosis reduces postoperative vomiting after surgery of the breasts. A prospective, randomized and blinded study. Acta Anaesthesiol Scand 1997;41(8):1028–32.

[34] Zeltzer LK, Dolgin MJ, LeBaron S, et al. A randomized, controlled study of behavioral intervention for chemotherapy distress in children with cancer. Pediatrics 1991;88(1):34–42.

[35] Pinnell CM, Covino NA. Empirical findings on the use of hypnosis in medicine: a critical review. Int J Clin Exp Hypn 2000;48(2):170–94.

[36] Redd WH, Montgomery GH, DuHamel KN. Behavioral intervention for cancer treatment side effects. J Natl Cancer Inst 2001;93(11):810–23.

[37] Watcha MF, White PF. Postoperative nausea and vomiting. Its etiology, treatment, and prevention. Anesthesiology 1992;77(1):162–84.

[38] Patterson DR, Jensen MP. Hypnosis and clinical pain. Psychol Bull 2003;129(4):495–521.

[39] Spiegel D. The mind prepared: hypnosis in surgery. J Natl Cancer Inst 2007;99(17):1280–1.

[40] Flory N, Salazar GM, Lang EV. Hypnosis for acute distress management during medical procedures. Int J Clin Exp Hypn 2007;55(3):303–17.

[41] Lang EV, Chen F, Fick LJ, et al. Determinants of intravenous conscious sedation for arteriography. J Vasc Interv Radiol 1998;9:407–12.

[42] Goubert L, Craig KD, Vervoort T, et al. Facing others in pain: the effects of empathy. Pain 2005;118(3):285–8.

[43] Singer T, Seymour B, O'Doherty J, et al. Empathy for pain involves the affective but not sensory components of pain. Science 2004;303(5661):1157–62.
[44] Watt-Watson J, Garfinkel P, Gallop R, et al. The impact of nurses' empathic responses on patients' pain management in acute care. Nurs Res 2000;49(4):191–200.
[45] Esdaile J. Mesmerism in India and its practical application in surgery and medicine Reissued as Hypnosis in medicine and surgery. New York (1957). London: Julian Press; 1846.
[46] Spiegel D, Detrick D, Frischolz E. Hypnotizability and psychopathology. Am J Psychiatry 1982;139:431–7.
[47] Astin JA. Why patients use alternative medicine. JAMA 1998;279:1548–53.
[48] Spiegel D, Bloom JR, Yalom ID. Group support for patients with metastatic cancer: a randomized prospective outcome study. Arch Gen Psychiatry 1981;38:527–33.
[49] Erickson MH, Rossi EL, Rossi SI. Hypnotic realities. New York: Irvington Publishers; 1976.
[50] Naparstek B. Successful surgery—health journeys, tape recording. Available at: www.healthjourneys.com/product_detail.aspx?id=29. Accessed February 1, 2008.
[51] Huddleston P. Prepare for surgery, heal faster. Cambridge (UK): Angel River Press; 1996.
[52] Wain HJ. Reflections on hypnotizability and its impact on successful surgical hypnosis: a sole anesthetic for septoplasty. Am J Clin Hypn 2004;46(4):313–21.
[53] Rausch V. Cholecystectomy with self-hypnosis. Am J Clin Hypn 1980;22(3):124–9.
[54] Barabasz AF. Whither spontaneous hypnosis: a critical issue for practitioners and researchers. Am J Clin Hypn 2005;48(2–3):91–7.

Hematol Oncol Clin N Am 22 (2008) 727–736

HEMATOLOGY/ONCOLOGY CLINICS
OF NORTH AMERICA

Incorporating Complementary and Integrative Medicine in a Comprehensive Cancer Center

Moshe Frenkel, MD*, Lorenzo Cohen, PhD

Integrative Medicine Program, The University of Texas M.D.
Anderson Cancer Center, 1515 Holcombe Boulevard, Unit 145, Houston, TX 77030, USA

With the increasing interest in complementary and integrative medicine (CIM) as an adjunct to conventional therapy among patients and families affected by cancer, more medical clinics and cancer centers are trying to address public interest and demand by providing CIM services. Despite a few attempts to organize and incorporate CIM services into the current health care system, the best method for integrating CIM therapy has not yet been established. Unfortunately, there is also limited research on the integration of CIM into conventional cancer care.

In 2002, the Federation of State Medical Boards in the United States developed and adopted new guidelines for the use of complementary and alternative therapies in medical practice [1]. These guidelines include recommendations for state medical boards on how to educate and regulate physicians who use CIM in their practices. These guidelines also suggest an organizational structure for integrating accepted standards of care with legitimate medical uses of CIM. In the United Kingdom, reports of CIM integration were mentioned in the British Medical Association's guide for general practitioners on referring patients to CIM practitioners, which is an important source of information on referral patterns [2]. This document relates primarily to the British health care system, however, and is narrow in scope. The guide does not address important universal issues related to the integration process, such as knowledge on CIM efficacy and safety; provider referral patterns and appropriate patient triage; CIM provider selection and accreditation; and communication-related issues between patients, CIM providers, and physicians.

Most of the information on integrative medicine centers in the United States comes from the recently established centers that are affiliated with hospitals around the country. The experience from these centers is informative [3]. Sporadic initiatives in primary care are mentioned, but few relate to the integration process for CIM [4–7].

*Corresponding author. *E-mail address*: mfrenkel@mdanderson.org (M. Frenkel).

0889-8588/08/$ – see front matter
doi:10.1016/j.hoc.2008.04.002

A few theoretic models of CIM integration were recently published. Leckridge [8] proposed a consumer-supplier model based on varying degrees of regulation and a patient-centered model emphasizing a shift in the balance of power from the professionals to the patients. Boon and colleagues [9] proposed seven models of team-oriented health care practice along a continuum that moves from nonintegrative parallel practice to fully integrative practice, with multiple situations that differ in philosophy, structure, process, and outcomes. The nonintegrative parallel practice side of the continuum is characterized by independent health care practitioners and each practitioner performs his or her job within his or her formally defined scope of practice. In this situation, the CIM practitioner has no connection or communication with the conventional health care professional. The fully integrative approach to patient care consists of an interdisciplinary, nonhierarchical blending of both conventional medicine and CIM health care and support. Fully integrated practice is based on a specific set of core values that include treating the whole person, assisting the innate healing properties each person possesses, promoting health and wellness, and preventing disease. Fully integrated practice requires consensus building between all health care professionals (conventional and nonconventional) and the patient, mutual respect, and a shared vision of health care that permits each practitioner and the patient to contribute their particular knowledge and skills within the context of a shared, synergistically charged plan of care [9]. Mann and colleagues [10] similarly described seven different models of integration, ranging from the informed individual practitioner to the more complex interdisciplinary models that involve various levels of integrated patient management through a partnered arrangement. All these models bring a theoretic basis to the process of integration relating to knowledge, credentials, location, and communication patterns. The main weakness of all these descriptions of team health care practices, however, is that they are based on theoretic assumptions and not derived from scientific data or systematic studies.

The integration of CIM practices, therapies, and beliefs with conventional health care practices can expand available treatment options, improve patient and provider satisfaction, better balance the deficiencies in each system, and lead to improved therapeutic outcomes [10]. Despite the interest of the general public, increased number of CIM practitioners, and enhanced interest among physicians to learn more about CIM, the process of integrating CIM into the conventional setting is slow [11] because of multiple barriers and obstacles. These obstacles include financial disincentives [12–15]; fear or concern with legal issues [12,16–18]; communication gaps between CIM providers, conventional health care staff, and conventional physicians [19]; identifying CIM providers and integrating them into the system; and lack of access to proper education about CIM [12,20–22]. Other obstacles include conventional system resistance, differences in beliefs about healing, limited information on clinical outcomes, and lack of experience and knowledge on how to overcome these obstacles [10,12,21–31]. Observing practices and identifying what can be learned from those practices helps identify ways to overcome these obstacles and barriers so the integration process can become successful [10].

THE PROCESS OF INTEGRATING COMPLEMENTARY AND INTEGRATIVE MEDICINE IN CANCER CARE: A MODEL IN A COMPREHENSIVE CANCER CENTER

The best process for incorporating CIM into conventional health care is complex and not well defined. The experience is limited and there is currently no consensus on the best model. Moreover, when the disease being treated is cancer, the situation becomes even more complex. All the factors mentioned previously are relevant in a cancer setting and other factors also enter the situation. Additional issues relevant in a cancer setting are the already high use of extreme CIM practices, intense fear of death, experiential sense of existential crisis, high degree of uncertainty, complex treatments, often unclear disease course and prognosis, and possible interactions between CIM and conventional treatments. These are just a few factors among many that make CIM use in cancer care even more problematic.

Little has been written about integrating CIM into cancer care because the field of integrative oncology is in its infancy. Described next is a model that has gradually developed in the past few years of integrating CIM services in a major comprehensive cancer center based on previous experience with integrating CIM in other primary care settings.

The University of Texas M.D. Anderson Cancer Center is located in Houston, Texas, on the campus of the Texas Medical Center. M.D. Anderson is devoted exclusively to cancer patient care, research, education, and prevention. The doctors and researchers at M.D. Anderson are renowned for their ability to treat all types of cancer, including rare or uncommon diseases, and patients with challenging prognoses. The institution is one of the nation's original three comprehensive cancer centers designated by the National Cancer Act of 1971 and is one of 39 National Cancer Institute–designated comprehensive cancer centers today. More than 79,000 people with cancer receive care at M.D. Anderson annually, and more than 27,000 of them are new patients. About one third of these patients come from outside Texas. More than 11,000 patients participated in therapeutic clinical research exploring novel treatments in Fiscal Year 2006, making it the largest such program in the nation.

Close to a decade ago, a survey conducted at M.D. Anderson revealed that 83% of patients used some form of CIM [32]. Because of patient interest and demand, in 1998 M.D. Anderson opened the Place... *of wellness*, the first onsite facility at a National Cancer Institute Comprehensive Cancer Center to provide CIM therapies to patients and caregivers who wanted to explore complementary therapy options. Over the next decade, this small clinical setting gradually expanded from a small facility to a large operation. Currently, more than 40 unique programs are offered in two locations on M.D. Anderson's campus, with an average of 145 complementary therapies and program opportunities conducted each month, including acupuncture, massage therapy, nutrition, music therapy, meditation, yoga, and aromatherapy. In 2006, more than 8500 people attended classes, with 55,000 contacts. Approximately 45% of the therapies and classes are related to stress reduction and mind-body therapy. Patients are referred to the services at Place... *of wellness* by their health care team or they self-refer, except for acupuncture or massage. Other than acupuncture and massage, all services are free of charge. Although most programs are held at one of the two locations on the main campus of M.D. Anderson, some programs are available at the bedside and in different clinical centers.

The CIM programs are facilitated by over 50 M.D. Anderson faculty, staff, and community practitioners who are credentialed in their respective areas of expertise. A comprehensive process is used to credential CIM practitioners to incorporate their expertise into the care practices provided to patients, which has been described in detail elsewhere [33].

A key to the success of this program is that it grew gradually with full institutional support. It was critical in the early stages to involve senior leadership at the institution and ensure that they supported integrative oncology at M.D. Anderson. It was also important to involve key stakeholders in any area overlapping with integrative medicine to ensure that the programs expanded in a collaborative and not competitive fashion. It was also critical to involve the institutional legal group and institutional compliance to ensure that all programs followed institutional requirements and regulations. It is also critical during the founding and growth phases to involve patients in the decision-making process, because it is being built for them and the available programs must meet their needs. As the program grew and became an indispensable service for patients and caregivers, it became clear that more formalized physician-led consultation services were needed to meet patient needs.

Individual Complementary and Integrative Medicine Consultations

Over the years there was an increased interest and patient demand for CIM. In addition, both patients and health care professionals at M.D. Anderson were in need of a more formalized integrative medicine consultation. As CIM use increased it became clear that a physician with extensive knowledge in CIM in oncology was needed to develop a consultation service to guide patients in the proper use of CIM related to their disease process.

In 2007, a new integrative medicine clinic opened through the Supportive Care Center at M.D. Anderson. This clinic started by providing an individual CIM consultation service to patients. The consultation is offered to patients who want advice on integrating CIM into their care or if the physician thinks that a consultation would benefit the patient. The basic principles of patient-centered care guides the consultation including (1) paying attention to the patient's psychologic and physical needs; (2) allowing the patients to disclose their concerns; (3) conveying a sense of partnership; and (4) actively facilitating patient involvement in the decision-making process [34].

The consultation addresses the main concerns that patients have about CIM use during and after their cancer treatment. During the consultation, patients can share concerns and expectations about CIM and the clinic staff addresses these issues in a way that empowers patients during their cancer journey. The consultation involves discussing CIM use with the patient and their family and facilitating an educated use of different complementary medicine modalities.

Using reliable sources of information and complementary therapies individualized to each patient helps reduce the uncertainty and anxiety experienced by patients and their families during and after cancer therapy. A physician can make a consultation request through an easy online process that is similar for all other consultation requests made in the institution. The patient and their caregivers, family members, or significant others are seen in a consultation room designed specifically to provide a healing environment that uses soft lighting, relaxing music, aromatherapy, and specially designed furniture.

The consultation consists of an assessment and review of the patient's medical history and a physical examination. The physician determines what conventional treatments have been tried, failed, or rejected because of safety, quality of life, cost, or another issue. The following questions are considered during this portion of the consultation: Is the patient coming for consultation during radiation therapy or chemotherapy or receiving other forms of conventional therapy? What types of conventional therapies are being used? What are the current physical and emotional problems that the patient and their caregivers are experiencing? What are the main reasons for the consultation? Patients sometimes come to the consultation with high expectations for cure or marked improvement in their condition by using CIM, while ignoring some important signs and symptoms that first require the attention of a conventional approach. For example, a patient may want to try an herb or supplement to counteract their extreme fatigue; however, the fatigue could be caused by severe anemia, which could require a blood transfusion.

A discussion of the patient's psychologic-social-spiritual perspectives is a crucial component of the consultation that helps the clinic staff to establish rapport with the patient and their family members or significant others. During this stage, the physician identifies the patient's beliefs, fears, hopes, expectations, and experience with CIM; explores what levels of support the patient relies on from their family, community, and friends; acknowledges the patient's spiritual and religious values and beliefs, including the patient's views about quality of life and end-of-life issues; and seeks to understand how all of these factors impact the patient's health care choices.

The consultation also involves an integrative medicine evaluation, and after a review of the patient's current and previous CIM use, the physician advices on how to combine different complementary medicine treatments into the current treatment plan. Important questions include: What types of therapies were used? How were the therapies used? Why were they used? A discussion of the patient's previous experience with CIM and current expectations from CIM is necessary for devising a plan for CIM use that the patient and their family can actively participate in developing.

Because of the intense emotions, deep belief systems, and often existential crises disclosed during the consultation, the consultations can become extensive and require empathy, compassion, and active listening from the physician requiring at times a prolonged visit of 60 to 120 minutes. The consultation process may also involve one or all of the following:

- A literature search to determine the state of the evidence for certain treatments when needed
- A review of what is found from previous research related to the scientific literature about integrative treatment for the patient's specific condition (eg, what is known on integrative therapies for advanced liver tumors)
- A review of what the patient is taking (which therapies have support in the scientific literature, and which do not? If there is support, what kind of evidence [randomized trials, single arm trials, case reports, epidemiologic data, and so forth])
- A review of the possible interactions with current medications, with pharmacist involvement, if needed
- A review of the patient's diet and supplements, with nutritionist involvement, if needed
- A discussion of the physician's current knowledge or findings with the patient and their family members or significant others
- A mutually agreed on plan
- Involvement of the Place... of wellness and referrals to CIM therapies and classes that the physician thinks will benefit the patient and their family
- A follow-up visit, usually after 6 to 12 weeks, to review progress or if any new issues have arisen (Fig. 1).

Each consultation is fully documented in the patient's electronic medical record, and each practitioner who works with the patient at the institution can review the details of this consultation process. If any questions arise, any member of the health care team can easily reach the integrative medicine physician by pager, telephone, or email.

The Integrative Medicine Consultation Clinic

At present, the integrative medicine clinic staff consists of an integrative medicine physician, holistic nurse, and integrative nutritionist. A team of CIM practitioners and selected conventional medicine professionals support the clinic operation with advice by telephone, emails, and a weekly meeting where an extended integrative medicine team meets to discuss complex situations and unique patient concerns.

The holistic nurse gathers basic history information from the patients before the physician's evaluation and the administrative and specific nursing tasks. The holistic nurse also provides "emotional first aid" when necessary by compassionately and empathetically listening and, at times, using integrative techniques, such as relaxation, imagery, reflexology, and therapeutic touch, to help patients and their family members, partners, and caregivers, especially when the patients are in distress. In addition, the nurse is the main contact

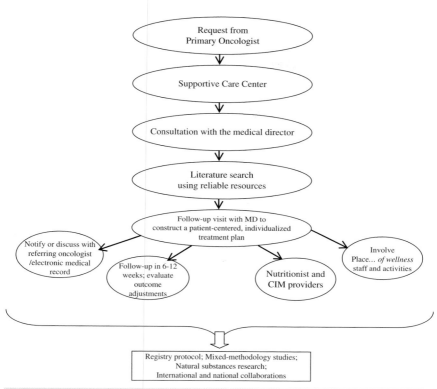

Fig. 1. Integrative medicine consultation process.

person if a patient requires additional information between visits. If the nurse cannot address the questions, they are brought to the physician's attention.

The integrative nutritionist, a registered dietician, plays a critical role in supporting the evolving clinical services. The nutritionist's main tasks include evaluating, assessing, and addressing patients' individual nutritional needs and concerns; involving family members in the process; evaluating diets and nutritional supplements the patient is already using; defining misconceptions and controversies related to diet, nutrition, supplements, and other natural products and developing strategies and guidelines to address them; and assessing research related to nutrition and health relating to each patient. The nutritionist also identifies nutritional therapies for the prevention and management of disease and evaluating the efficacy of nutritional interventions; explains the rationale and use of nutritional and dietary supplements; identifies food and nutrient interactions; educates and counsels patients regarding dietary change; and produces patient education material that addresses patients' concerns that were disclosed in the integrative medicine clinic. When applicable, the nutritionist addresses the issue of "stress and nutrition," evaluates and participates in developing research related to nutrition and integrative cancer care, and participates in educational forums to educate patients, caregivers, and medical staff on issues related to nutrition and integrative cancer care.

Once a week, the integrative medicine team meets to discuss complex situations and unique patient concerns, brainstorm on possible solutions that can benefit the patient and their caregivers, and discuss specific incidents as they relate to each member's experience in providing integrative care in the institution.

The team consists of professionals employed at M.D. Anderson who have experience in conventional approaches to cancer care and knowledge and experience in integrative oncology. The team includes:

- Information specialists who have experience researching reliable information sources related to CIM therapies involved in caring for patients with cancer
- A nutritionist with expertise in monitoring diets and nutritional supplements and the use of food as a medicinal element in the treatment of cancer
- A holistic nurse who coordinates care and provides the missing link in between visits
- A pharmacist with expertise in complementary substances, including nutritional supplements, vitamins, herbs, and other natural products, and the interactions these substances may have with each other and with conventional medications
- Mind-body specialists who can suggest appropriate techniques, including music therapy, yoga, meditation, relaxation, expressive arts, and more, that can be used to reduce stress and anxiety; these specialists may also address spiritual issues
- Massage therapists who have experience with manual therapies that can help with relaxation, stress reduction, and improved symptom management
- An acupuncturist who has experience managing patients' pain, discomfort, and other symptoms resulting from illness or the side effects of conventional treatment
- A physical therapist or occupational therapist who can add a point of view on physical activity and rehabilitation
- A natural substance expert (ethno pharmacist) with expertise in herbs, foods, vitamins, and minerals that adds a unique viewpoint on various nutritional supplements

A large proportion of patients that come for the integrative medicine consultation are also referred for further CIM classes and treatments to Place... *of wellness.*

The interest in this consultation service was quite surprising and resulted in a quick increase in the number of clinical consultation sessions from two to four sessions a week in 2 months of operation, with only a minimal marketing effort. By March 2007, the clinic was working at full capacity at 4 half days per week, with over 200 visits from patients by the end of 2007. Most of the patients were satisfied with one visit that answered most of their concerns. On average, one third of the patients felt the need to come for further follow-up visits to address their concerns.

SUMMARY

The process of incorporating CIM with conventional medical care is a complex process. The experience is limited and there is currently no consensus regarding the integration of CIM into conventional care. Trying to address this process in cancer care is even more complicated. A model for integrating CIM into the conventional cancer care in a comprehensive cancer center requires cooperation from the key institutional stakeholders and a gradual infiltration into the system in a staged programmatic fashion. The clinical model for integrative care requires a patient-centered approach with attention to patients' concerns and enhanced communication skills. In addition, CIM practitioners' and conventional practitioners' involvement and working together in developing this integration process are essential. This process requires tremendous team effort, institutional culture change, trust and open communication between all members of the health care team, and major support from the institutional leaders.

Acknowledgments

This work was not possible without the individual contribution of all the Supportive Care Center staff, the Integrative Medicine Program administrative and educational staff members, the educational resources available at M.D. Anderson, and the Place. . . *of wellness* staff, facilitators, and practitioners.

References

[1] New model guidelines for the use of complementary and alternative therapies in medical practice. Altern Ther Health Med 2002;8(4):44–7.
[2] General, practitioners, and committee, referrals to complementary therapists: guidance for GP's. 1999; London.
[3] Weil A. The significance of integrative medicine for the future of medical education. Am J Med 2000;108(5):441–3.
[4] Frenkel MA, Borkan JM. An approach for integrating complementary-alternative medicine into primary care. Fam Pract 2003;20(3):324–32.
[5] Elder C. Integrating CAM into practice: the KP northwest story. The Permanente Journal 2002;6:57–9.
[6] Paterson C. Complementary practitioners as part of the primary health care team: consulting patterns, patient characteristics and patient outcomes. Fam Pract 1997;14(5):347–54.
[7] Paterson C. Primary health care transformed: complementary and orthodox medicine complementing each other. Complement Ther Med 2000;8(1):47–9.
[8] Leckridge B. The future of complementary and alternative medicine: models of integration. J Altern Complement Med 2004;10(2):413–6 [review].
[9] Boon H, Verhoef M, O'Hara D, et al. From parallel practice to integrative health care: a conceptual framework. BMC Health Serv Res 2004;4(15).
[10] Mann D, Gaylord S, Norton SK. Integrating complementary and alternative therapies with conventional care (the convergence of complementary, alternative and conventional health care: educational resources for health professionals). University of North Carolina at Chapel Hill. Program on Integrative Medicine 2004;35.
[11] Kessler RC. Long-term trends in the use of complementary and alternative medical therapies in the United States. Ann Intern Med 2001;136:262–8.
[12] White House Commission on Complementary and Alternative Medicine policy WHCCAMP, final report 2002; Washington, DC.

[13] Pelletier KR, Astin JA. Integration and reimbursement of complementary and alternative medicine by managed care and insurance providers: 2000 update and cohort analysis. Alternative Therapies 2002;8(1):38–48.

[14] Pelletier KR, Astin JA, Haskell WL. Current trends in the integration and reimbursement of complementary and alternative medicine by managed care organizations (MCOs) and insurance providers: 1998 update and cohort analysis. Am J Health Promot 1999;14(2): 125–33.

[15] Canfield D, Faass N. Perspective: funding sources for an alternative medicine clinic. In: Faass N, editor. Integrating complementary medicine into health systems. Gaithersburg (MD): Aspen; 2001. p. 122–5.

[16] Cohen MH. Legal issues in complementary and integrative medicine: a guide for the clinician. Med Clin North Am 2002;86:185–96.

[17] Cohen MH, Eisenberg DM. Potential physician malpractice liability associated with complementary and integrative medical therapies. Ann Intern Med 2002;136(8):596–603.

[18] Cohen M. Legal issues in integrative medicine. 2005: National Acupuncture Foundation. 90.

[19] Crock RD, Jarjoura D, Polen A, et al. Confronting the communication gap between conventional and alternative medicine: a survey of physicians' attitudes. Altern Ther Health Med 1999;5(2):61–6.

[20] Berman BM. Complementary medicine and medical education. BMJ 2001;322(7279): 121–2.

[21] Frenkel M, Ben Arye E. The growing need to teach about complementary and alternative medicine: questions and challenges. Acad Med 2001;76(3):251–4.

[22] Konefal J. The challenge of educating physicians about complementary and alternative medicine. Acad Med 2002;77(9):847–50.

[23] Barrett B, Marchand L, Scheder J, et al. Bridging the gap between conventional and alternative medicine. J Fam Pract 2000;49(3):234–9.

[24] Druss BG, Rosenheck RA. Association between use of unconventional therapies and conventional medical services. JAMA 1999;282(7):651–6.

[25] Eisenberg DM, Cohen MH, Hrbek A, et al. Credentialing complementary and alternative medical providers. Ann Intern Med 2002;137(12):965–73.

[26] Hess D. Complementary or alternative? Stronger vs. weaker integration policies. Am J Public Health 2002;92(10):1579–81.

[27] Kingston S. The assessment of clinical skills for practitioners of complementary medicine. Complement Ther Med 1996;4:202–3.

[28] Astin JA, Marie A, Pelletier KR, et al. A review of the incorporation of complementary and alternative medicine by mainstream physicians. Arch Fam Med 1998;158(21):2303–10.

[29] Faass N. Integrating complementary medicine into health systems. Gaithersburg (MD): Aspen Publications. 763; 2001.

[30] Jain N, Astin JA. Barriers to acceptance: an exploratory study of complementary/alternative medicine disuse. J Altern Complement Med 2001;7(6):689–96.

[31] Mootz RD, Coulter ID, Hansen DT. Health services research related to chiropractic: review and recommendations for research prioritization by the chiropractic profession. J Manipulative Physiol Ther 1997;20(3):201–17.

[32] Richardson MA, Sanders T, Palmer JL, et al. Complementary/alternative medicine use in a comprehensive cancer center and the implications for oncology. J Clin Oncol 2000;18(13):2505–14.

[33] Baynham-Fletcher L, Babiak-Vazquez AE, Cuello D, et al. Credentialing complementary practitioners in large academic cancer center. J Soc Integr Oncol, in press.

[34] Mead N, Bower P, Hann M. The impact of general practitioners' patient-centredness on patients' post-consultation satisfaction and enablement. Soc Sci Med 2002;55(2):283–99.

Hematol Oncol Clin N Am 22 (2008) 737–753

HEMATOLOGY/ONCOLOGY CLINICS
OF NORTH AMERICA

Ethical Issues in Integrative Oncology

Eran Ben-Arye, MD[a,*], Elad Schiff, MD[b,c], Ofra Golan, LLD[c,d]

[a]Complementary and Traditional Medicine Unit, Department of Family Medicine, Faculty of Medicine, Technion-Israel Institute of Technology, Clalit Health Services, 6 Hashahaf Street, Haifa 35013, Israel
[b]Department of Internal Medicine, Bnai-Zion Hospital, 47 Golomb Street, Haifa 31048, Israel
[c]Department for Complementary/Integrative Medicine, Law, and Ethics, International Center for Health, Law, and Ethics, Haifa University, Har HaCarmel, Haifa 31905, Israel
[d]Unit for Genetic Policy and Bioethics, Gertner Institute for Epidemiology and Health Policy Research, Tel Hashomer 52621, Israel

I ntegrative oncology is a term conceptualized in recent years based on a significant attitude change of conventional medical systems toward complementary and alternative modalities of care. In the early 1990s, the abbreviation CAM (complementary and alternative medicine) was applied by medical scholars in relation to the broad spectrum of medical systems and techniques that were considered at the time outside the boundaries of conventional medicine. Often, researchers, clinicians, and medical educators defined CAM on an exclusion basis—that is, therapies that are not practiced in health care and are not taught in medical schools [1]. This definition reflected the unfamiliarity of the American Academy and health system with leading CAM modalities (eg, herbal, traditional, homeopathic, and other CAM medical systems) compared with the extensive tradition, knowledge, experience, clinical research, and integration of CAM in western and central Europe, China, India, and other third world countries. The establishment of the National Institutes of Health Office of Alternative Medicine in 1992 and the National Center of Complementary Alternative Medicine (NCCAM) in 1997 marked a notable shift in American awareness to the importance of CAM and positioned the United States as a dominant contributor to global CAM research, medical education, and clinical practice. Today, the public and the scientific community acknowledge CAM more as "complementary" rather than "alternative" to mainstream medicine. The reasons for this attitude are multifaceted and relate to the extensive use of CAM among the general United States population (about 60%) [2] and its ramifications on the doctor–patient relationship [3], along with the expansion of evidence-based CAM research and the ongoing

All authors contributed equally.

*Corresponding author. Clalit Health Services, Haifa and Western Galilee District, 6 Hashahaf Street, Haifa 35013, Israel. *E-mail address*: eranben@netvision.net.il (E. Ben-Arye).

0889-8588/08/$ – see front matter
doi:10.1016/j.hoc.2008.04.009

integration of CAM within the medical curriculum in many United States medical schools [4,5]. In the last decade, the term *complementary* is gradually shifting to *integrative-based medicine* [6]. The concept of integrative medicine is based on the following foundations: a patient-centered biopsychosocial-spiritual holistic approach, an obligation for evidence-based research and practice, and a commitment for the integration of CAM within conventional medical settings based on collaborative MD and non-MD CAM and conventional practitioners' multidisciplinary teamwork [7].

The concept of integrative oncology relates to the fruitful dialog emerging between CAM scholars, oncologists, family practitioners, and other health care providers who envision an extended and holistic patient-centered approach to oncology care [8]. This movement is based on the paradigm change in conventional oncology moving from a strict biomedical orientation toward a biopsychosocial-spiritual context as manifested in concepts of palliative care, quality-of-life improvement, spirituality, and narrative-based medicine [9]. Thus, the interest in CAM modalities relevant to cancer care is not limited to questions of efficacy and safety but includes their impact on patients' suffering, coping, thinking, feeling, willing, and creativity. Moreover, CAM modalities such as mind-body, Chinese, and anthroposophic medicine may not only alleviate specific pain or gastrointestinal symptoms but may also induce an outlook change in patients who have cancer through seeking the meaning of disease in their life or accepting disability and death. This dual commitment of integrative oncology to a medical humanistic approach and to an evidence-based foundation imposes considerable ethical concerns. Health care providers, including dual practitioners (MD and CAM), may often struggle with ethical conflicts concerning the integration of CAM treatment in oncology settings due to lack of sufficient evidence to support its efficacy, safety, and potential interactions with chemo- and radiotherapy. In addition, they may find ethical difficulties such as the inability to talk freely with their colleagues or patients in cases in which they sense an inappropriate level of invasive treatment that contradicts their personal or professional health-belief model. These ethical considerations are becoming more and more important as CAM is acknowledged by governmental agencies (eg, the Office of Cancer Complementary and Alternative Medicine of the National Cancer Institute) and integrated within leading oncology care hospitals (eg, MD Anderson in Texas, Sloane-Kettering Memorial Hospital in New-York, and more).

In many aspects, ethical considerations in integrative oncology are not remarkably different from other fields of medicine [10,11]. The four principles of general biomedical ethics include beneficence (obligation to seek the patient's good), nonmaleficence (avoiding harm), respect for autonomy, and justice [12]. In 2005, the Institute of Medicine (IOM) published an extensive in-depth report on CAM, which included a chapter on the ethical framework for CAM [13]. The IOM report suggested five ethical values, including (1) beneficence (interpreted also as social commitments to public welfare, including access provision to the best information available on CAM efficacy); (2) protection and nonmaleficence—a commitment to *primum non nocere*, which includes not only safety issues but also "respecting divergent cultural beliefs and creating an emotionally safe environment for the discussion of CAM"; (3) respect for patient autonomy (and consumer choice); (4) recognition of medical pluralism ("a moral commitment of openness to diverse interpretations of health and healing"); and (5) public accountability, which includes "a sensitivity to the complex needs and desires of multiple constituents within the public sector." Cohen [14], a leading scholar in CAM bioethics, argued that physicians may experience conflict between their evidence-based orientation and the patient's interest in CAM and suggested they balance the major bioethical principles "on a case-by-case basis." Furthermore, Cohen and colleagues [15] suggested a framework of seven considerations for drawing ethical conclusions, including severity of illness; curability; invasiveness and safety of conventional treatment; evidence of CAM efficacy/safety; the patient's knowledge; understanding and acceptance of the risk/benefit of CAM and of conventional treatments; and degree of the patient's persistence/intention to use CAM. Rosenthal and Dean-Clower [16] discussed the integration of CAM in hematology/oncology and addressed (from practical, ethical, and legal perspectives) the need for patient–physician communication regarding CAM, especially concerning CAM–conventional treatment interactions. Robotin and Penman [17] added to the ethical discussion of integrative oncology the need to determine the practitioner's knowledge level of CAM treatments to not only provide CAM risk/benefit information but also skillful referral to qualified CAM practitioners and the ability to "remain involved in a patient's care." The significance of this last theme is further highlighted by the findings of a qualitative study from Israel and Australia: some of the patients who decided to stop active conventional treatment for cancer were CAM users who looked for spiritual dimensions in their care and wished to be more active in their own healing [18].

This article presents a case study from three different points of view: the clinical outlook, the patient's narrative, and her physician's narrative. The authors contemplate the three outlook angles and characterize the patient's and the physician's ethical conflicts in the integrative setting. The authors also suggest a practical ethical framework for integrative physicians who may transform ethical constraints into a communication tool.

CASE STUDY—CLINICAL OUTLOOK: THE 55-YEAR-OLD MULTIPLE MYELOMA PATIENT

Mrs. D is a 55-year-old woman who was in general good health until she felt pain in her right hip. She made an appointment with her family physician whom she acknowledges as "holistic" and skillful in conventional and "natural medicine." The family physician prescribed a local nonsteroidal anti-inflammatory gel, which only partially alleviated the pain. At the next appointment, the physician suggested treatment with a homeopathic remedy, which did not help. Subsequently, Mrs. D was referred for radiography of the hip, which showed a lytic lesion. Further evaluation included cytogenetic and fluorescent in situ hybridization examinations that showed no pathology, and a bone marrow biopsy that showed foci of plasma cells. A probable diagnosis of solitary plasmacytoma or multiple myeloma was established.

Following radiotherapy, the patient developed severe limping for which her orthopedic oncologist prescribed clodronate and a glucosamine/chondroitin combination, with some relief. At that time, the patient turned to her family physician seeking a "healing" complementary plan in the realm of anthroposophic medicine. The family physician referred Mrs. D to curative eurythmy (anthroposophic movement therapy). He also consulted with anthroposophic oncologists and hematologists concerning the efficacy and safety of treatment with subcutaneous injections of the herb *Viscum album* (European mistletoe). Following these consultations, a recommendation to start *Viscum* treatment was provided. Mrs. D, however, declined *Viscum* treatment but expressed gratitude to her physician for making the consultation effort. She started feeling better due to the eurythmy treatment and the natural remedies prescribed by her son.

A year later, a high load of free light kappa chains was detected in the patient's blood. The hematologist suggested vincristine, adriamycin, and dexamethose (VAD) chemotherapy for probable myeloma. The patient declined therapy saying the hematologist's worldview was narrow and incongruent with her own. The patient, however, continued to receive care from the orthopedic oncologist and her family physician, who asked her to continue with follow-up visits to the hematologists.

Six months later, the patient began suffering from severe upper back pain. She referred herself to a massage practitioner and homeopath, who offered some relief. At that time, her family physician ordered a CT scan, which revealed multiple lytic lesions of the spine consistent with her primary disease. After further consultation with her family physician, the patient was referred to another hematologist, and is now receiving VAD chemotherapy.

CASE STUDY—PATIENT'S OUTLOOK: THE WOMAN WHO FACES ILLNESS

Mrs. D is a 55-year-old mother living with her spouse. The couple has two children in their late 20s: one son is studying abroad and the other son is still living with the parents but considers leaving home. Mrs. D teaches art and is closely related to anthroposophic philosophy, which views spirituality as an integral part of the human body and mind. Based on this health-belief model, Mrs. D and her family had chosen a few years ago to join the public clinic of a family medicine specialist trained in complementary therapies, including anthroposophic medicine. Before her illness, Mrs. D's primary expectation of her family physician was "to listen to her" ("be present and attentive") and to suggest advice and "natural" remedies if possible and "conventional" drugs only if absolutely indicated.

Mrs. D faces the grave diagnosis of multiple myeloma by experiencing symptomatic hip pain rather than comprehending her ailment as "a form of cancer." She is grateful to receive local radiation therapy from the orthopedic oncologist who complements the treatment by prescribing both conventional (clodronate) and complementary (glucosamine/chondroitin) therapies. Following completion of the radiation treatment, Mrs. D asks her family physician to build a complementary rehabilitation program based on anthroposophic medicine and to collaborate with the orthopedist and hematologists (the conventionalists). Mrs. D is choosing to accept her family physician's advice concerning eurythmy treatment, which is related to her reliance on anthroposophic medicine and her interest in art. At the same time, she is receiving herbal treatment recommended by her son, who feels the need "to actively do something" for his mother.

After a few weeks, Mrs. D suffers less limping and feels that the "acute" phase is behind her. Although she asked her family physician to consult with some well-known anthroposophic physicians worldwide, she feels that the appropriate way to advance her healing is not by referring "outwardly" to cancer medications (conventional or anthroposophic) but rather "inwardly" by "being myself."

A year later, Mrs. D is facing the hematologist's more definitive diagnosis of multiple myeloma and the need for chemotherapy treatment. Mrs. D feels that the hematologists' language, metaphors, and health-belief model are completely dissimilar to her own. Although Mrs. D acknowledges the hematologists as professional and dedicated to patients, she feels that she cannot accept this disease-oriented and spiritually lacking approach. She decides to cancel further appointments with any hematologist and to rely only on follow-up of her orthopedic oncologist and family physician, although they clarify that they are less competent than hematologists for managing her myeloma.

Six months later, Mrs. D is facing the recurrence of pain but decides to first refer to "alternative" practitioners rather than her family physician, who eventually refers her to a CT scan that reveals the severity of her illness. Mrs. D now faces not only the objective grave diagnosis but also the need to return to the hematology arena, which she characterizes as "nonhealthy and poisonous" and contradictory to her health-belief model. Mrs. D is fully aware of her critical condition but still asks her family physician to find alternative treatments to chemotherapy and bone marrow transplantation. Mrs. D and her husband meet their family physician and are persuaded by his decisiveness regarding necessity of conventional treatment and lack of reasonable alternative options. They talk about options in choosing hematologists who may be more receptive toward Mrs. D's beliefs. Mrs. D feels a gradual ability to start chemotherapy treatment.

CASE STUDY—MRS. D'S FAMILY PHYSICIAN'S OUTLOOK: A PHYSICIAN IN BETWEEN ALTERNATIVE AND INTEGRATIVE ONCOLOGY

Dr. B is a 44-year-old physician (specialist in family medicine) who also has training in herbal, homeopathic, and anthroposophic medicine. Dr. B is interested in evidence-based CAM and views his work in a public family medicine clinic in an integrative context, combining a biopsychosocial family medicine approach with complementary therapies.

Dr. B is medically familiar with Mrs. D and her family and has addressed acute minor ailments (eg, sore throat) and more in-depth interventions, such as depression of one of the family members, for several years. When Mrs. D presented with mild right hip pain (her myeloma presenting symptom), Dr. B offered a simple therapy that was also used as a diagnostic trial. Dr. B prescribed a nonsteroidal anti-inflammatory gel complemented by a homeopathic remedy. After a few days of persisting pain, Dr. B referred Mrs. D to radiographic examination followed by CT scan to complete a full diagnostic process.

When the diagnosis of a lytic lesion was evident, Dr. B referred Mrs. D to the hematology and orthopedic oncology departments for treatment. In the following months, Mrs. D updated her family physician with medical letters from the orthopedic oncologist and hematologist and asked his assistance in various administrative procedures. At this time, Dr. B was less involved in his patient's care and experienced the role of a "secondary player" in the overall medical plan. Following the radiation treatment, Mrs. D approached her family physician to seek advice concerning a healing program. Dr. B, who recommended integration of anthroposophic treatment along with hematology follow-up, was gaining back his central role in Mrs. D's management. A referral of Mrs. D to anthroposophic movement therapy (eurythmy) was part of a structured anthroposophic treatment plan that relates to (1) a general anthroposophic approach to cancer and to the individual characteristics of Mrs. D's illness, (2) Mrs. D coping with her disease, and (3) supporting spiritual development. Dr. B also raises the possibility of adding *Viscum* injections to the treatment. *Viscum* serves as a core treatment element in anthroposophic oncology along with varied art therapies; however, evidence is lacking for the efficacy and safety of *Viscum* in the treatment of myeloma. Hence, Dr. B seeks expert opinions from anthroposophical physicians and shares with Mrs. D the dilemma on potential efficacy versus unknown safety data. The patient asks him to be her guide in treatment decision and acknowledges scientific uncertainty. The consultation with anthroposophic oncologists worldwide is concluded with a recommendation for *Viscum* treatment but the patient declines this treatment. At this time, Mrs. D and Dr. B experience a new communication gap. Mrs. D is moving toward a more "alternative" health-belief model, leaving her family physician in a relatively conventional role. This gap is evident for nearly a year until a new crisis appears. During the meetings that take place in his office, Dr. B shares with Mrs. D his worries of inappropriate hematologic follow-up but affirms his commitment to her medical treatment "even if we do not agree about the same health beliefs."

Dr. B is made aware of Mrs. D's new onset of pain only after weeks of alternative massage and homeopathic treatments prescribed by other practitioners. The persistence of pain worries Mrs. D and her family who ask for urgent tests, which confirm the diagnosis of widespread disease. The meeting with Mrs. D and her husband marks another milestone in the relationship with Dr. B who is again asked "to navigate the ship in stormy water" and to recommend the hematologist and the hospital where Mrs. B would receive what Dr. B regards as "unavoidable chemotherapy." During the following meetings, Dr. B and Mrs. D discuss how Mrs. D can prepare herself for the journey of chemotherapy and bone marrow transplantation and how this experience may become an integral part of her spiritual growth.

FOLLOW-UP OR RELATIVE CONCLUSION OF THE CASE STORY

Mrs. D and Dr. B met again at the end of the second VAD chemotherapy treatment. Mrs. D's face was shining and smiling. She described the dramatic metamorphosis she had to face in her health belief and spirituality to accept the need for chemotherapy. She described the difficulty of accepting the "non-self-treatment" of chemotherapy into her inner spiritual sense of "self," regarded by her as the "I" or the "ego organization." She said that the acceptance of the chemotherapy had also influenced the way she perceived herself, her life, and her family. Dr. B asked Mrs. D about her difficulties and suffering and suggested the metaphor of a plant growing outwardly from the solid and humid earth to the light and air. Mrs. D replied with her enchanting smile. A sense of growth and birth was present in the room as Mrs. D left to start her third cycle of outward and inward therapy.

DISCUSSION

The story takes place in a primary care clinic that combines conventional and CAM approaches in an integrative worldview. As within ancient Greek theater, we are presented with the three main characters: the patient (Mrs. D), the family physician (Dr. B), and the disease (multiple myeloma). One can easily identify the other secondary players: the husband (and the sons), the orthopedic oncologists, the two hematologists, and the alternative practitioners. One can even sympathize with some of the characters or feel uneasiness with the way Mrs. D or Dr. B relates to them. Unlike a Greek tragedy, however, integrative medicine is not based on the dichotomy of sympathy and antipathy or conventional and alternative but relates to the notion of relativity. The concept of relativity in integrative medicine means that one quality (eg, black) is not absolute but defines—and is defined by—another quality (ie, white). As with the Chinese philosophy of yin and yang, the two "opposite" qualities not only complement each other but also define each other and generate one another. Thus, Dr. B, the family physician who seeks an integrative model of care, is not in opposition to the alternative practitioners or the conventional hematologists. The evolution of the therapeutic dialog between Dr. B and Mrs. D illustrates the relativity of the two characters. The narratives of the doctor and the patient emphasize this relativity. Thus, along one phase of the story, Mrs. D appears "more alternative" relative to Dr. B, "the conventionalist," whereas in other phases, Dr. B may be characterized as "too alternative" by Mrs. D, the hematologist, or the reader. The ethical meaning of being an integrative practitioner is not merely restricted to the beneficence-to-maleficence ratio but also includes the skills and ability to act as a therapist who can move on the scale between the conventional and the alternative poles. The concept of respect for patient autonomy demands another ability of integration: to move on the scale between the pole of flexibility and sympathy (understand the patient even if you do not agree with her/him) and the other pole of stiffness and antipathy (to support the patient in her/his uncertainty like a flagpole in a stormy sea). The authors suggest that in this case study, ethical concerns and dilemmas are not restricted to the integrative family physician but also to the patient, the alternative practitioners, and the conventional hematologists/oncologists. Table 1 highlights the ethical dilemmas of these four groups in accordance with the five ethical values of the IOM report.

ETHICAL ISSUES CONCERNING DR. B'S PERSPECTIVE AS AN INTEGRATIVE PHYSICIAN

Possible Conflicts Among the Values of Professionalism, Beneficence, and Nonmaleficence

What is considered a sufficient level of evidence regarding the efficacy and safety of *Viscum* injections to recommend it to Mrs. D? How ethical is it to prescribe CAM therapies merely on the basis of clinical judgment or expert opinions from anthroposophic physicians?

Patient Autonomy Versus the Commitment of Protection and the Obligation of Nonabandonment

What are the implications of Mrs. D's choice of Dr. B as her primary care provider in terms of treatment decisions concerning multiple myeloma treatment? Should Dr. B fully respect Mrs. D's "alternative" health belief? To what extent is he obligated to patients who have extreme "alternative" health beliefs?

The Ethical Commitment to Medical Pluralism

How should Dr. B build a bridge between their two perspectives and how will this gap influence the communication with her CAM practitioners, orthopedic oncologist, and hematologists?

Medical Pluralism Versus the Duty of Competency

In light of the value of medical pluralism, to what extent is Dr. B responsible for the coordination of CAM therapies and therapists? Is the level of responsibility in correlation with his personal or professional scope of education and practice?

Public Accountability Versus Patient Autonomy

From a public accountability viewpoint, should society point to Dr. B and his fellow integrative physicians to be those who specialize and care for alternative-oriented patients like Mrs. D, serving as the "CAM gatekeepers" of society? Who is responsible for the treatment of ultra-alternative patients who view conventional treatment as contradictive to their health belief?

ETHICAL ISSUES CONCERNING MRS. D'S PERSPECTIVE AS PATIENT

Should alternative practitioners (ie, massage therapist and non-MD homeopath) inform Mrs. D that conventional medicine is not in their scope of practice? Could lack of such a declaration cause a delay in her diagnosis and treatment of widespread myeloma lesions? Can these therapies cause direct harm?

The Difference Between Respect of Autonomy and the Promotion of Autonomy and the Possibility of Conflict with the Principle of Beneficence

Should integrative physicians and CAM practitioners ask patients like Mrs. D to sign an informed consent form? Does informed consent respect, promote, or restrict the patient's autonomy?

The Value of Medical Pluralism

Who should be committed to collaborating among the integrative family physician, CAM practitioners, oncologists, and hematologists? In a world of medical pluralism, who would be willing to be the patient's gatekeeper and case manager?

Patient Autonomy Versus Public Accountability

Do Mrs. D and other CAM proponents have the ethical right to demand CAM inclusion in the national health/health maintenance organization budget just because they use CAM or identify with its health philosophy?

ETHICAL ISSUES CONCERNING THE ALTERNATIVE PRACTITIONERS' PERSPECTIVE

The Commitment to Protect Patients

Can CAM practitioners be fully aware of the risks of CAM? Are they fully aware of the possible benefits and risks of conventional treatment? To what extent do they have substantial knowledge concerning CAM–conventional medicine interactions?

The Principles of Autonomy and Nonmaleficence

Can CAM practitioners working outside mainstream medicine endanger the patient and her autonomy by not informing her of the full consequences of CAM "outcomes" and the avoidance of conventional therapies?

The Commitment to Public Accountability

To what extent should CAM practitioners be committed not only to their patients but also to the public and the medical health system?

ETHICAL ISSUES CONCERNING CONVENTIONAL HEMATOLOGISTS' AND ONCOLOGISTS' PERSPECTIVES

The Commitment to Protection Versus Medical Pluralism

To what extent are Mrs. D's hematologists and oncologists aware of the risk/benefit ratio of CAM and possible interactions with conventional therapy? Is it

Table 1
Ethical dilemmas of integrative physicians, alternative practitioners, conventional physicians and patients in light of the five ethical values of the IOM report

Ethical value	Integrative physician	Patient	Alternative practitioners	Hematologists, oncologists
Beneficence and Protection	To what extent is a low level of efficacy/safety evidence sufficient to recommend a treatment to a patient who has a serious illness? How ethical is it to prescribe CAM on the basis of clinical judgment, expert opinion, personal experience, or "logic" of traditional/CAM schools of medical thought?	Should the patient be informed that conventional medicine is not in the scope of CAM practitioners? Can this cause false or late diagnosis and induce harm?	Can CAM practitioners be fully aware of the risks of CAM? Is the CAM practitioner fully aware of the possible benefits and risks of conventional treatment? To what extent should the CAM practitioner know or inquire about CAM–conventional interactions?	To what extent are physicians aware of the risk/benefit ratio of CAM and possible interactions with conventional therapy? Do they have an ethical obligation to study CAM research published in mainstream medical journals?
Patient autonomy	Does a patient's initial choice in alternative or integrative care justify full respect of his/her will?	Do the two ethical commitments of patient autonomy and informed consent necessarily interact in favor of the patient? Do patients have a "real" free choice when they receive spiritual and nonscientific treatment?	Can CAM practitioners working outside mainstream medicine endanger patient autonomy?	To what extent should physicians respect the patients' agenda? Should a physician continue therapy if he/she feels inability to respect patient's autonomy? To what extent should physician autonomy be considered?

Medical pluralism	Do integrative physicians have an ethical commitment only to their patients or should they be responsible and committed to the coordination of CAM therapies and therapists? To what extent should integrative physicians be committed to CAM medical systems that are out of their personal/professional scope of education and practice?	Who should be committed to the collaboration between the various medical schools of thought and be responsible for adequate physician–CAM practitioner communication? In a world of medical pluralism, who would be willing to be the patient's gatekeeper and case manager?	To what extent may CAM practitioners view their practice as the "real medicine" and collaboration with mainstream medicine as a necessary "politically correct" obligation? What is the scope of the commitment to medical pluralism in cases of a nonmutual relationship between the dominant and the nondominant practice? Should CAM practitioners be ethically committed to a dialog with their patient's physician?	To what extent should physicians rely only on scientific evidence-based data? Is commitment to medical pluralism a "necessary burden" or an opportunity to enrich physicians' communication skills and scope of practice and decrease physicians' burnout?
Public accountability	To what extent should the integrative physician be obliged to patients who have an extreme alternative health-belief model? Should the integrative physician be more committed to such patients as the "CAM gatekeeper" of the society?	Do patients have the ethical right to demand/oppose CAM inclusion in the national health/health management organization budget just because they use or do not use CAM?	To what extent should CAM practitioners be committed not only to their patients but also to the public? Should CAM practitioners' ethical commitment to public health influence their approach to self-regulation and CAM legal status?	How ethical is it to support, ignore, or avoid CAM consultation in a public medical institution? Should physicians expect health system administrators to "fill in" their gap in CAM knowledge?

ethical to offer CAM treatments not based on evidence (eg, the orthopedic oncologist who offered glucosamine treatment following radiation) just to "satisfy" Mrs. D's health belief? Do oncologists and hematologists have an ethical obligation to study CAM research published in mainstream medical journals?

The Commitments to Patient Autonomy Versus Medical Pluralism and Nonabandonment

To what extent do physicians need to respect Mrs. D's worldview? Should they continue to hold medical responsibility for her care even if they believe they are unable to respect her autonomy? To what extent should physician autonomy be considered?

Public Accountability

How ethical is it to support, ignore, or avoid CAM consultation in a public medical institution? Should physicians expect health system administrators to refer them to basic introductory courses in CAM or to advanced learning in integrative oncology? From an ethical point of view, should oncologists call for the establishment of integrative clinics in the oncology clinical service?

ANALYSIS OF A CHOSEN ETHICAL DILEMMA

All the questions just stated present ethical issues and concerns faced by the various parties involved in the care of the patient. Nevertheless, only some of the questions constitute an ethical dilemma because such a dilemma is, by definition, a conflict between two or more values or principles [19].

Such a conflict apparently rises in relation to one theme that is entwined in several concerns from the physicians' perspective—that of professionalism. The dilemma regarding the appropriateness of the treatment is "In what circumstances, if any, would it be ethically justifiable for a physician to compromise the requirement of scientific evidence in favor of other moral values?" This concern might be rephrased as a conflict between the principles of beneficence and nonmaleficence vis-à-vis those of respect for autonomy and medical pluralism.

The recommended way to deal with this dilemma is by using the risk framework suggested by Cohen and Eisenberg [20]. According to this framework,

> If evidence [concerning the CAM therapy] supports both safety and efficacy, the physician should recommend the therapy but continue to monitor the patient conventionally. If evidence supports safety but is inconclusive about efficacy, the treatment should be cautiously tolerated and monitored for effectiveness. If evidence supports efficacy but is inconclusive about safety, the therapy could still be tolerated and monitored for safety. Finally, therapies for which evidence indicates either serious risk or inefficacy obviously should be avoided and patients actively discouraged from pursuing such a course of treatment.

In the context of Mrs. D's case, the issue of appropriate treatment was raised by the family physician in relation to his decision to recommend treatment with *Viscum* injections. As to the quality of evidence of safety and efficacy of this treatment, despite extensive experience with this treatment in various cancers, there is no solid evidence about its use in similar circumstances but only data of potential efficacy and unknown safety. This situation seems to be defined as one in which "evidence supports efficacy but is inconclusive about safety" in which "the therapy could...be tolerated and monitored for safety." Such a decision should be made following consideration of the other six factors in the framework of Adams and colleagues [15] for risk-benefit analysis of CAM versus conventional medical treatment:

1. Severity and acuteness of illness
2. Curability with conventional treatment
3. Degree of invasiveness, associated toxicities, and side effects of conventional treatment
4. Degree of understanding of the risks and benefits of CAM treatment
5. Knowledge and voluntary acceptance of those risks by the patient
6. Persistence of the patient's intention to use CAM treatment

In the case of Mrs. D, the severity of the illness was high and, at that stage, there was no conventional treatment other than monitoring. The patient was willing to use CAM treatment, understood the potential consequences of the proposed treatment with *Viscum*, and acknowledged the scientific uncertainty thereof. In these circumstances, Dr. B's decision to offer *Viscum* was appropriate. For her own reasons, however, the patient decided to decline his recommendation.

The issue of appropriateness is further raised in relation to the orthopedic oncologist's prescription of glucosamine/chondroitin. From a CAM perspective, there was no indication or logic in prescribing this formula to Mrs. D following radiotherapy; however, there is no known risk from its use. According to the IOM's ethical framework for CAM, "when there is no evidence for or against a given CAM therapy, physicians can choose to tolerate and monitor or actively discourage use of CAM treatments" [13]. The authors believe that this recommendation refers to situations in which a patient requests a certain treatment that has no proven benefit but is not to be taken as support for physicians to suggest such a treatment.

Related to this is another aspect of professionalism—the issue of competency. This issue concerns not only which CAM treatments should be offered but also who should and should not be allowed to offer them. How far can physicians who are not qualified in CAM go to meet their patient's wishes to receive CAM treatments? The dilemma is that the doctor's commitment to respect the patient's autonomy and the commitment to medical pluralism may outweigh his/her primary duty for competency. A second reading of this apparent dilemma, however, suggests that such a value conflict is not ethically possible because competency is a sine qua non for practicing health care. The rule of *primum non nocere* outlaws any possibility of physicians practicing (unattended) a form of care in which they lack prior knowledge or experience unless it is done within properly authorized clinical research. Practicing with the intention to please a patient who wishes to have CAM treatment combined with a conventional one could never accord with respect for the patient or for medical pluralism. Such a behavior is an expression of disrespect to the patient's wish to be treated by CAM, because giving her an ineffective treatment is not what she wants and pretending that it should benefit her while there is no basis for such a presentation constitutes deception. It also does not accord with the commitment to medical pluralism: to prescribe a nonindicated therapy merely because it is categorized as CAM shows disrespect to CAM as though it were not a professional area and implies that "it's all placebo anyway."

Thus, under this analysis and with the helpful guidelines about CAM treatment decisions, it seems as if these dilemmas should not have been an issue in this case.

Yet the hard feelings that presented themselves in the form of the integrative family physician's dilemmas seem to have resulted from miscommunication with the patient. Dr. B spots his recommendation to use *Viscum* injections as the junction in which he might have taken the wrong direction. He is concerned about it despite doing what seems to be a dedicated search and taking thorough consideration, with a remarkable process of shared decision making with the patient. Had Dr. B been uncertain about this recommendation, he would probably have been relieved by Mrs. D's decision not to accept it. According to his narrative, however, after "the patient declines this treatment, Mrs. D and Dr. B experience a new communication gap." At the same time, the patient happily receives her conventional orthopedic oncologist's prescription for glucosamine treatment, which in her condition is no more than a CAM placebo, and an herbal treatment recommended by her son to answer his "need to do something" for her.

It is obvious that Dr. B, as an integrative physician, knew that the information he gathered from experts worldwide about the use of *Viscum* injections in the circumstances of this case was almost equivalent to scientific evidence, whereas the other treatments the patient was taking were medically useless, though not harmful. So, it is not the dilemma of professionalism that disturbs him, but it is clear from his story that he feels as though he had missed something in the management of this patient at that point. How come Mrs. D chose to reject Dr. B's recommendation and to loose contact with him after asking him to be her guide in this decision and expressing her gratitude to him for making the consultation efforts?

As seen from her narrative, the cause of Mrs. D's behavior was her perception of the "outward" versus "inward" healing process. As we can tell from the end of the story, Dr. B was capable of dealing with Mrs. D's perception of the healing process, but they did not touch this issue until a year and a half later. It turns out, as we can tell in hindsight, that what the physician could and probably should have done at that time was to ask the patient her reasons for declining the treatment. The reason he did not ask was probably because he had a real dilemma about the appropriateness of this treatment. Having that in mind, he might have assumed that Mrs. D's reasons to choose differently were those raised by him as considerations against this treatment, and he decided to respect her autonomy. Had he not held such a belief, he would have probably have asked the patient why, and a different story would have been told through these "sliding doors."

This analysis shows that struggling and dealing with an ethical dilemma might blur one's mind from looking for further aspects of the issue. The lesson from this case is that within doctor–patient relationships, communication is irreplaceable. If a patient decides to go against a physician's advice, the physician should always strive to discover the underlying reasoning for this decision. Asking why does not interfere with respect for the patient's autonomy, whereas assuming that you know why and guessing the patient's reasons can end with great surprises. The authors' concluding advice is to listen to patients not only because they may be guiding you toward their diagnosis and treatment but also because any ethical dilemmas of the encounters may unfold in their narratives.

SUGGESTED PRAGMATIC ETHICAL APPROACH TO MRS. D-LIKE PATIENTS IN THE INTEGRATIVE ONCOLOGY CONTEXT

The authors suggest a pragmatic ethical approach to patients who challenge their oncologist, family physician, CAM practitioner, or integrative physician. The concept of relativity discussed in this article means that we—patients and therapists alike—are moving on a scale between what seems to be contradictory elements. The "alternative" of today may be regarded as "conventional" tomorrow, and the dichotomy of black and white may turn to the "integration" of black seed within white that generates the white seed within black. Thus, absolute "truth"—like evidence-based medicine to the oncologist, holistic medicine to the CAM practitioner, or spirituality to a patient like Mrs. D—are in constant change on the scale between objectivity and subjectivity, anxiety and reassurance, "doing" and "being."

The authors suggest regarding the uneasy dialog with "noncompliant" and "troublesome" patients who hold alternative-oriented health beliefs as a "gift" that may open us to a new outlook on our own health-belief model and our ability to grow as therapists. Inasmuch as we learn clinical medicine from our patients, we may develop our communication abilities with patients (and with colleagues and ourselves) following meeting with them, "the other." The following suggestions may be useful to facilitate meeting with CAM-oriented patients from an ethical worldview in the oncology context:

- Observe the patient's subtext and note whether you recognize in yourself a sense of unease.
- Ask patients whether they feel any incongruence between their belief systems and the treatment suggested by other therapists/physicians or by you.

Consider asking patients specifically about their health beliefs and how they relate to their dilemmas.

- Contemplate and define your main ethical dilemmas and how your own health-belief model may influence them. Consider sharing your own dilemmas with the patient.
- Follow-up a discussion of safety and efficacy issues by further contemplating the meaning of these data (or the absence of solid evidence) by acknowledging medical pluralism and viewing different CAM and conventional health approaches.
- Inform patients about potential therapies from a beneficence and maleficence perspective and add a macroeconomic and public accountability perspective of what can be offered in private, public, or half-paid medical services.
- Conclude the discussion by asking the patient to define the appropriateness of the treatment strategy in terms of his/her wish to be involved, dominant, passive, assertive, or collaborative in the sacred space of the patient's and therapist's autonomy.

References

[1] Eisenberg DM, Kessler RC, Foster C, et al. Unconventional medicine in the United States. N Engl J Med 1993;328:246–52.

[2] Barnes P, Powell-Griner E, McFann K, et al. Complementary and alternative medicine use among adults: United States, 2002. Adv Data 2004;27(343):1–19.

[3] Ben-Arye E, Ziv M, Frenkel M, et al. Complementary medicine and psoriasis: linking the patient's outlook with evidence-based medicine. Dermatology 2003;207(3):302–7.

[4] Lee MY, Benn R, Wimsatt L, et al. Integrating complementary and alternative medicine instruction into health professions education: organizational and instructional strategies. Acad Med 2007;82(10):939–45.

[5] Wetzel MS, Kaptchuk TJ, Haramati A, et al. Complementary and alternative medical therapies: implications for medical education. Ann Intern Med 2003;138(3):191–6.

[6] Weil A. Integrated medicine imbues orthodox medicine with the values of complementary medicine. BMJ 2001;322:119–20.

[7] Bell IR, Caspi O, Schwartz GE, et al. Integrative medicine and systemic outcomes research: issues in the emergence of a new model for primary health care. Arch Intern Med 2002;162(2):133–40.

[8] Cassileth BR, Vickers AJ. High prevalence of complementary and alternative medicine use among cancer patients: implications for research and clinical care. J Clin Oncol 2005;23:2590–2.

[9] Deng GE, Cassileth BR, Cohen L, et al. Society for Integrative Oncology Executive Committee. Integrative oncology practice guidelines. J Soc Integr Oncol 2007;5(2):65–84.

[10] Vohra S, Cohen MH. Ethics of complementary and alternative medicine use in children. Pediatr Clin North Am 2007;54(6):875–84.

[11] Ernst E, Cohen MH, Stone J. Ethical problems arising in evidence based complementary and alternative medicine. J Med Ethics 2004;30:156–9.

[12] Tilburt JC, Miller FG. Responding to medical pluralism in practice: a principled ethical approach. J Am Board Fam Med 2007;20(5):489–94.

[13] Committee on the Use of Complementary and Alternative Medicine by the American Public. An ethical framework for CAM research, practice and policy. Complementary and alternative medicine in the United States. Institute of Medicine of the National Academies; 2005.

[14] Cohen MH. Legal and ethical issues in complementary medicine: a United States perspective. Med J Aust 2004;181(3):168–9.

[15] Adams KE, Cohen MH, Eisenberg D, et al. Ethical considerations of complementary and alternative medical therapies in conventional medical settings. Ann Intern Med 2002;137(8):660–4.

[16] Rosenthal DS, Dean-Clower E. Integrative medicine in hematology/oncology: benefits, ethical considerations, and controversies. Hematology Am Soc Hematol Educ Program 2005;491–7.

[17] Robotin MC, Penman AG. Integrating complementary therapies into mainstream cancer care: which way forward? Med J Aust 2006;185(7):377–9.

[18] Kacen L, Ariad S, Madjar I, et al. Patients deciding to forgo or stop active treatment for cancer. European Journal of Palliative Care 2005;12(3):113–6.

[19] Beauchamp TL, Childress JF. Principles of biomedical ethics. 3rd edition. Oxford University Press; 1989. p. 4.

[20] Cohen MH, Eisenberg DM. Potential physician malpractice liability associated with complementary and integrative medical therapies. Ann Intern Med 2002;136(8):596–603.

Hematol Oncol Clin N Am 22 (2008) 755–766

HEMATOLOGY/ONCOLOGY CLINICS
OF NORTH AMERICA

Remarkable Recoveries: Research and Practice from a Patient's Perspective

Marc Ian Barasch

PO Box 3444, Boulder, CO 80305, USA

Twenty-some years ago I was diagnosed with papillary carcinoma of the thyroid. The standard treatment—the removal of the gland and its replacement by a daily pharmaceutic—struck me at the time as radical and alarming. Before agreeing to the procedure, I asked my surgeon if such tumors were ever known to regress.

"Never," he said, enumerating the mortal dangers of wishful thinking and blind hope. Clearly he found me naïve, and I was—about the sinister depredations of cancer, surely, but also about the degree of (understandable) medical skepticism about the body's self-healing capacity when it comes to cancer's dire domain.

At the time, I was editing a magazine that covered the nascent stirrings of complementary and alternative medicine. I had seen instances where serious disease had resolved in ways that seemed outside the conventional medical paradigm. I noted that such patients had often adopted rigorous alternative regimens, pursued disciplines of mind and body, and made other life-changes to which they (if not their doctors) ascribed their cures.

Their methods usually had no trial-verified therapeutic value (suggesting their conditions were either misdiagnosed, self-resolving, or the result of nonreplicable healing modalities). Nonetheless, I had set out into the unknown, using such crude maps as I could find. I began eating fresh vegetables and whole grains, eliminating red meat, fried foods, refined sugar, and excess salt. Office overtime also went by the wayside. I started on a regimen of yoga and meditation, gulped vitamin supplements, and focused on people and pursuits that made me happy.

Despite my illness, I began to feel better than I had in years. But after several months of this, feeling like a pioneer forging too deep into uncharted territory,

---

Portions of this article are drawn from Hirschberg C, Barasch MI. Remarkable recovery. New York: Riverhead Books; 1995.

E-mail address: marcbar1@mac.com

0889-8588/08/$ – see front matter
doi:10.1016/j.hoc.2008.04.011

I opted for a thyroidectomy. I was startled, however, by my postoperative biopsy report: during those months, the volume of the tumor had shrunk by nearly half from its original scanned measurement.

This is not to claim that my ad hoc approach would have effected a cure. The occurrence of so-called "spontaneous remission" of cancer is rare, with estimates ranging from 1 in 60,000 to 1 in 100,000 (though some investigators maintain it is grossly underreported) [1]. Still, my experience led me to spend nearly a decade studying unusual survivors, wondering if the stories of such "outliers" might contain key insights into the healing process.

It is a path trodden by investigators with better credentials. When Dr. Steven Rosenberg, the former Chief of Surgery of the National Cancer Institute (NCI), was a junior surgical resident, he treated a 51-year-old war veteran, one Mr. DeAngelo, for an infected gall bladder. Yet Mr. DeAngelo, with what Rosenberg would later remember as "an aura of secret triumph," regaled him with a story the young doctor assumed was a product of the befuddlements of old age and alcohol: Mr. DeAngelo insisted he had once had terminal stomach cancer with liver metastases and it had just . . . gone away.

Digging out the original pathology report, Rosenberg confirmed, the man had once been diagnosed with terminal cancer. In the course of the gall bladder operation, Rosenberg took the time to carefully probe the man's liver for the metastases he was sure he would find. But there were none. "I rushed out of the operating room," Rosenberg later wrote. "This didn't seem possible. There had been only four documented cases—not four a year in the United States, but four, ever, in the world—of spontaneous and complete remission of stomach cancer." Mr. DeAngelo, he realized, "presented a mystery of ultimately enormous dimensions" [2]. Dr. Rosenberg went on to devote a substantial portion of his career to seeking ways to augment the body's immune response. While at the NCI, he famously devised an experimental treatment for advanced cancer using cells engineered to produce tumor necrosis factor [3].

A colleague of mine once attended a medical seminar that veered into a discussion of the odd case of Mr. DeAngelo, an alcoholic who polished off several quarts of bourbon a week. A doctor had interjected: "Did the guy quit drinking after they told him he had cancer?" Told no, he had asked, amid his colleagues' swelling laughter, "Well, then, what *kind* of whiskey did he drink?"

His question wasn't entirely facetious. What had happened? Dr. Rosenberg's bare-bones case report provides no clues: "No evidence of tumor or other masses could be found in the abdomen. No adenopathy could be palpated" [2]. To sift through the medical annals of such cases is to be confronted by accounts dry to the point of dessication. We are told next to nothing about who these people actually were, what occurred in their journey, or what they think was essential to their cure.

REMARKABLE RECOVERY

Could the human side of these unusual cases yield hints about what causes such radical departures from normal disease progression? It was in pursuit of this question that my coauthor, researcher Caryle Hirshberg, PhD, and I wrote *Remarkable Recovery*. The book grew out of our probing of some 60 medically verified cases of unexpectedly long survival or complete cure of advanced disease, mostly cancer. We chose the term "remarkable recovery" to counter the more common term "spontaneous remission," a nomenclature implying such cases so elude scientific understanding they can only be relegated to a mystery zone.

We proposed a more embracing definition, including not just instances of outright disappearance of incurable pathology, but cases where healing mechanisms other than treatment might be surmised to have caused exceptional outcomes: living in equilibrium with disease for unexpectedly long periods of time, or radically delayed progression, or recovery following merely palliative procedures. We took care to verify each case. Our source materials were medical records, case reports, articles in referenced journals, patient and physician interviews, and psychosocial questionnaires.

Looking at these cases, it was clear many were the products of multifactorial processes that would not lend themselves to the fine parsing of Occam's Razor. The phenomenon of remarkable recovery may be produced by a cascade of biologic response modifiers we do not fully understand, including alternative medicines, quirks in the genetic make-up of the host or the tumor, mind-body mechanisms, psychosocial factors, or—most challengingly—all of the above.

PSYCHOSOCIAL INTERVENTIONS

There has been much controversy over whether psychosocial intervention can affect disease progression. Frequently cited in its favor is a 1989 study by Dr. David Spiegel, which found that women with metastatic breast disease who received group therapy were more likely to be alive 18 months after diagnosis than a control group. However, several subsequent studies have failed to bolster this finding. Typical was a 2007 study, in *Psychooncology* [4], of the impact of supportive-expressive group therapy (SEGT) on survival in 485 women with advanced breast cancer. The trial found that although SEGT did improve quality of life and afforded protection against depression, there was no prolonged survival (median was 24.0 months in SEGT, and 18.3 months in controls).

Another 2007 article in *Cancer* [5] by Dr. Spiegel, detailing his 14-year study of 125 women with metastatic breast cancer, created a stir when his results failed to replicate his prior study. Women placed in group therapy in the new study had survived an average of 30.7 months, compared with 33.3 months for the control group. "Group therapy not a boost to cancer survival after all," summarized a headline in the *San Francisco Chronicle*. "Psychologic support doesn't extend life for most breast patients" [6].

Behind the word "most," however, lay a finding of potential significance. A small subset of women with estrogen-negative breast cancer showed markedly better survival times with group therapy: 30 months versus 9 months for those who did not get therapy. The reason, Spiegel speculates, is that medical treatments for estrogen-positive breast disease have improved to such a degree (ie, hormonal treatments such as aromatase inhibitors) that psychotherapy provided little additional boost for survival. But in the case of estrogen-negative breast cancer, where treatment has not shown similar advances, the psychosocial intervention of group therapy seemingly made a difference.

It will take follow-up studies to determine if this result is borne out. But the animating question in Dr. Spiegel's work remains: How can physicians maximize the healing resources of their cancer patients? Do such resources even exist, or are the mechanisms of psychoneuroimmunology or biospsychosocial medicine too subtle—or chimerical—to substantially alter the course of disease? That is, do the patient's thoughts, emotions, and social relationships have genuine clinical significance beyond improving attitudes and making patients subjectively "feel better"? It is a question with profound implications for therapeutic design and for the patient's own journey.

BIOLOGIC MODIFIERS

Still, do such hard-to-quantify factors even need to be invoked? Various physiologic mechanisms and endogenous biologic response modifiers have been flagged as potentially relevant to cancer regression [7], including increased blood flow to (or elevated temperature at) the tumor site, actions by neuropeptides, changes in the body's biochemical "terrain," mobilization of immune factors, and genomic anomalies in host or tumor.

Everson and Cole [8] reported cases where people recovered after a mere biopsy, indicating a possible rousing of the immune system to combat tumors. Some recovered following transfusions of plasma and blood, hinting at the existence of blood-borne components that might react against the deadly interloper. Others had regressions after infections and high fevers. In the late nineteenth century, Dr. William Coley discovered a terminal sarcoma patient who had fully recovered following a severe streptococcal infection of the skin. Through trial and error, Coley devised a combination of streptococcal bacteria that reliably produced fevers of 104 degrees or more when injected at tumor sites, leading to unusual rates of remission. Coley [9] eventually documented a nearly 50% 5-year or more survival rate in 210 cases of soft-tissue sarcomas after induced infections and fever. However, as one researcher told us, "With Coley, tumor necrosis factor was only one short-lived piece of a cascade of effects orchestrated within the system. I'm not sure you can ever isolate some single active ingredient in the lab" [10].

DIET

This problem of isolation applies even more to changes in diet frequently reported by remarkable recoveries. These run the gamut from eating large quantities of meat to switching to entirely vegetarian diets (one woman who had an unexpected healing of malignant melanoma ate "nothing but grapes" [11]). Harold Foster [12], who reviewed 200 cases of remarkable recovery, found that nearly 88% reported making substantial dietary changes, "usually of a strict vegetarian nature," before their healing. But were these causative or concomitant? Retrospective studies of nutritional methods (eg, the so-called Gerson method [13] that features coffee enemas and copious quantities of carrot juice) have yielded intriguing findings but no acceptable level of proof.

MIND-BODY MODALITIES

What of possible mind-body modalities? In a January 2008 *New York Times* article, the cancer specialist Dr. Jerome Groopman wrote: "[D]espite several decades of concerted research in the field of psychoneuroimmunology, to my scrutiny no robust effects of meditation or other relaxation techniques that could combat illnesses like cancer or AIDS have been identified" [14].

Is this a fair statement, or are there mechanisms whereby such practices might play a role in the healing process? The pathways of psychoneuroimmunology, for example, may be startlingly precise. The *International Journal of Neuroscience* published an almost eerie experiment in "voluntary modulation of neutrophil adhesiveness" [15]. Students were taught self-hypnosis and visualization techniques, then given a description of the neutrophil's special functions and properties, focusing on the immune cell's ability to adhere. Subjects were told to devise their own personalized visual imagery to attempt to increase this property of stickiness. (One student, for example, imagined her neutrophils as Ping-Pong balls with honey oozing out, causing them to stick to whatever they touched.)

After two weeks of such training, saliva and blood samples were compared with those obtained before the experiment had begun. The samples were analyzed for neutrophils and other immune components: monocytes, lymphocytes, and platelets. There was no difference in any of the cell counts before and after. The only statistically significant change was that the neutrophils' ability to stick to foreign objects had increased.

A 1997 study of the effect of relaxation and guided imagery on the parameters of host defenses in women with advanced breast disease revealed increases in lymphokine activated killer (LAK) cell activity, and increased the total number of T cells (CD2+), mature T cells (CD3+), and activated T cells (CD25+). The intervention also reduced the circulating levels of tumor necrosis factor-alpha, though the clinical significance of these changes in terms in tumor biology could not be determined. Investigators also observed that the more vivid the imagery, the higher the natural killer (NK) and LAK cells' activity [16]. In a later prospective randomized, controlled trial by the same investigators—this one with of a group of 96 women with newly diagnosed large or locally advanced breast cancer—imagery ratings were positively correlated with clinical responses.

But the investigators also noted, "The problem with univariate analyses is that the different variables are often themselves intercorrelated: what we really want to find out is which variables are genuinely *independent* predictors of survival" [17].

MULTIFACTORIAL HEALING

One case I studied, a man named Peter Hettel [11], speaks volumes about the difficulty of ferreting out such "independent predictors," even as it suggests unconventional factors contribute to outcome. Hettel had been diagnosed at MD Anderson Cancer Center with an immunoblastic sarcoma in his sinus. The mass was debulked with laser surgery, but quickly began to grow back. The recommended treatment—removal of the sinus and pituitary gland, radiation, and possible blindness as a side effect—was refused by the patient.

Among other things, Hettel had devised a vivid set of visualizations: "I'd imagine white immune cell bunny rabbits feasting on fields of orange cancer carrots, which increased [the rabbits'] energy and sex drive, which made them make more bunnies who were also hungry to eat more cancer." One morning months later, Hettel recalls, "I couldn't find enough carrots for all my rabbits. I thought, 'Gee, I hope my bunnies are all right'" Not long after that, he had a vivid dream in which he was standing in a "cave of flesh" that had "big, pink, bulbous stalactites hanging down. . .[T]here was an earthquake, and . . . they crashed down from the roof to the floor."

A week later, while doing a yoga exercise, Hettel had an eruptive nosebleed. Running to the sink, he says, "I began to spit up what seemed like pieces of pink rubber eraser." Probing the roof of his mouth with his tongue, he was shocked to find a hole instead of the tumor's familiar protrusions. The doctor who had followed the case confirmed Hettel's story: "It was as if his body had rejected a foreign object, like a transplant rejection . . . I can't account for it, other than he seemed to change his living habits dramatically, adopted a take-charge attitude instead of just giving up. He began doing what he deeply wanted to do."

Hettel tried a variety of other markedly nontraditional modalities, as is often the case with remarkable recovery, where patients tend to mobilize every possible healing resource at their disposal, not worrying much about whether one or the other was the most "active ingredient." In addition to his visualizations, Hettel adopted a stringent health food diet laced with liberal quantities of carrot juice, and took up yoga and Zen meditation. He met a therapist who taught him alleged techniques for "neurologic repatterning." Her therapy also encouraged "self-love," producing episodes in which, Hettel reported, long-ignored emotions poured out and left him "mewling like a baby." A week before his tumor was expelled, he had a highly emotional argument with his father and "for the first time in my life . . . I just openly and honestly expressed my anger toward him."

IMMUNE RESPONSE AND EMOTIONS

Is what a psychiatrist would call "emotional catharsis" relevant to the healing process? Candace Pert, codiscoverer of endorphins, suggests: "Since immune cells have neuropeptide receptors, the biochemistry of emotion is mediating the migration of natural killer cells through the body." Because tumor cells also have such receptors, emotions, she suggests, may mediate their movements as well. Studies of potential negative biologic response modifiers—the immunosuppressant effects of stress, for example—also imply that emotions could be relevant to cancer progression. Other investigators urge considering not only how stress affects the immune surveillance that helps govern tumor survival, but how stress contributes to "somatic mutation and genomic instability ... It is possible that a sharper focus on other relevant biological processes such as increases in DNA damage, alterations in DNA repair, and inhibition of apoptosis, may explain more of the variance in disease outcomes" [18].

Is it possible, then, that states of relaxation or joy or emotional release would disinhibit apoptosis and promote DNA repair? It is provocative to wonder if one implication of psychoneuroimmunology is that many things are "medicine": could encouraging words from a physician, a loving relationship, a strong emotion, a vivid image all produce physiologic cascades that can influence disease outcomes?

A valid critique is sometimes lodged that such formulations may contribute to a "blame the victim" paradigm. "If I'm not getting well," a patient might reason, "I must not be trying hard enough." Patients may blame themselves for not cultivating the "right" attitudes or behaviors to affect the blind machinations of biology.

At the same time, properly framed, patients may be encouraged to develop coping strategies more conducive to general health and happiness, though these necessarily will vary from person to person. Investigator Lydia Temoshok [19] has suggested, for example, that the most positive factors in health maintenance are what she dubs the "Three Cs": control, commitment, and challenge. But for another person, it might be cantankerousness, compassion, and congruence. Still, of all the candidates for a "fourth C," I would firmly nominate "connection."

SOCIAL CONNECTION

Time after time, strong social connection has been prominent in cases of remarkable recovery: enduring marriages, devoted friendship, indestructible love. Many of these patients were able to mobilize social networks. Some reported that just one person's encouragement—whether a friend, a therapist, a doctor or nurse, or social worker—sustained them in their struggle against horrendous odds and formed the pivot point of healing.

The great majority of remarkable recoveries we studied had been married over 20 years, and 41% had been married over 30 years [11]. Studies have found that married persons live longer, "with lower mortality for almost every major cause of death, in comparison with single, separated, widowed, or divorced persons." Conversely, in one study of more than 27,000 cancer cases, it was found that unmarried persons had markedly poorer rates of survival [20].

In one study of leukemia patients preparing to undergo bone marrow transplants, 54% of those who said they had strong emotional support from their spouses, family, or friends were still alive after 2 years, while only 20% of those who said they had little social support had survived [21]. Concludes one recent study: "The link between personal relationships and immune function ... is one of the most robust findings in psychoneuroimmunology" [22].

The effect of social relationships may be traceable down to the cellular level. A recent (2005) study in the *Journal of Clinical Oncology* on the impact of social support and similar factors in ovarian cancer patients examined the relationship among distress, social support, and NK cell activity, peripheral-blood mononuclear cells, ascitic fluid, and tumor-infiltrating lymphocytes. The conclusion: "Psychosocial factors, such as social support and distress, are associated with changes in the cellular immune response, not only in peripheral blood, but also at the tumor level" [23]. The implications are profound: strengthening loving, supportive ties with others may be a vital therapeutic modality.

ISSUES IN RESEARCH AND APPLICATION

How can a factor like love or community be applied in a treatment regimen? How can any of these foregoing observations be applied? Whether or not a more extensive study of remarkable recovery produces legitimate (ie, replicable) therapeutic strategies with consistent and measurable results, increased study would surely yield suggestions for therapeutic design that augments not only the patient's will to live, but his or her joy in living.

Mind-body therapies are often portrayed in the literature as self-palliative, adjunctive, and complementary, but rarely as contributive to cure. Many physicians continue to view them as acceptable indulgences so long as they are harmless and the patient remains fully compliant with a standard treatment regimen. The possibility that such modalities might help drive the healing process itself is infrequently acknowledged. Observations of remarkable recovery may mandate we broaden the definition of "medicine" to include biopsychosocial factors that positively impact what Norman Cousins [24] once dubbed the "healing system" (which he defined as "a grand orchestration ... enabling human beings to meet a serious challenge").

It seems especially important to encourage physicians to publish their cases of remarkable recovery in referenced medical journals so that a true epidemiology of this phenomenon can emerge. The study of the odd, the unexpected, the hard-to-find and difficult-to-quantify has always been the challenge and glory of medicine. (The study of autoimmune disorders, for example, crucially advanced our knowledge of immunology.) But there has been scant methodologic study of remarkable recovery, not in small part because of how infrequently these cases are reported in the literature. This is not necessarily a reflection of their rarity, but a reluctance to write up these anomalies [25].

As suggested earlier, the scarcity of reports also stems from the lack of an appropriately broad definition that includes unexpectedly long survival, recoveries that were treated conventionally yet "shouldn't have happened," unusual recoveries resulting from a combination of conventional and alternative treatment.

A REMARKABLE RECOVERY REGISTRY?

Most reports contain precious little information about the individuals who are their subjects. Attempting to locate the actual patients behind the often-sketchy descriptions, I was surprised to discover how many doctors had lost track of their exceptional patients entirely. How can the scattered data on the subject be retrieved from its orphaned status in medicine? A Remarkable Recovery Registry modeled on (or perhaps even included within) the National Cancer Institute's Tumor registry might be a cornerstone.

New methods of interviewing and reporting are also needed. Each patient's unique characteristics may be as vital as his or her physiologic measures. Some of this information might be best obtained from a support person, whether family member, nurse practitioner, or social worker, likely to be familiar with the dimensions and details of the person's life. The patient's account of his or her experience, often dismissed as merely subjective, could also be considered as a source of data, particularly in the context of "the healing system."

By re-examining current therapeutic strategies in the context of possible mind-body factors brought to light in remarkable recovery, the testing of new medical protocols could be enhanced to the benefit of patients as well as medical treatment and education. The picture of the spectrum of self-repair could be broadened. Adding psychosocial assessments to intake procedures could lead to individualized treatment models. Gathering and analyzing solid data on remarkable recovery would give the concerned physician a means to provide "ethical hope" to even terminal patients. If remarkable recovery contains a social dimension, then placing focused attention on social support would become an essential component of medical treatment.

Are there genetic or other biologic anomalies in remarkable recovery patients? In *Remarkable Recovery*, we cite the case of a Seattle man who experienced a spontaneous regression of bronchogenic carcinoma [11]. The man's inquisitive physician, Dr. Bell, who wrote up the case twice for the *American Journal of Surgery*, incubated some of the man's lymphocytes and placed them in a Petri dish with another patient's lung cancer cells. While putting one patient's white cells in proximity to another's cancer cells would normally have little effect, Dr. Bell noted with surprise that his patient's leucocytes reduced the cancer cells' colony formation by more than half [26].

A Remarkable Recoveries registry would have a tumor bank and a plasma bank. A rigorous analysis of tissue and cells of enough individual cases could lead to a wealth of biologic information. With the advent of genomic testing and tools for cloning rare biologic factors, medical science is in a unique position to make groundbreaking discoveries about unique tumor-host mechanisms based on remarkable recovery cases.

Along with any insights into mechanisms of cure, cases of remarkable recovery have much to teach us about optimum ways to address the full spectrum of cancer patient needs. Should not all medical students learn skills that could help their patients mobilize the psychologic, emotional, and spiritual resources that may be a form of medicine? One survey showed that 90% of 649 oncologist respondents believed that attitudes of hope and optimism, a strong will to live, confidence in the doctor, and emotional support from family and friends had been of significant benefit to treatment [26].

A SOURCE OF HOPE

I was recently contacted by a woman, Karen Dennis (Karen Dennis, unpublished manuscript, 2008, quoted with permission), who had a well-documented remarkable recovery (from metastatic carcinoid cancer of the ampulla of vater). Her case may exemplify a model of doctor and patient working together to maximize all the healing resources at their mutual disposal. Dennis's journey ran the gamut from conventional treatment, to homeopathy, to cutting edge experimental chemotherapy, to a radical surgery opposed by five of six surgeons on her hospital tumor board. When, despite heroic medical efforts during an 11-year period, her metastases returned, she had decided to refuse further treatment and pursue a range of alternatives.

Dennis reports that "she struck a bargain" with her primary care physician, asking for his support in abandoning oncology and promising that if or when she became symptomatic again, she would submit to whatever diagnostic work he felt appropriate. He assented and, she reports, wrote her an unusual prescription:

> You have my permission to NOT accept your diagnosis.
> You have my permission to NOT accept your prognosis.
> Permission to be selfish and celebrate the miracles in your life.

This, Dennis says, "turned out to be the most compliant I had ever been with a treatment plan." When, 4 years later, she had her first CT scan since making her "compliant" decision, there was no evidence of disease. Her surgeon, Dr. John E. Niederhuber, who had in the interim become director of the National Cancer Institute, wrote her a letter that could serve as a template for how physicians might relate to such remarkable cases.

"I do not have a ready explanation for the miraculous recovery you have experienced," he wrote. "Because of cancer's complex nature, and the uniqueness of each individual affected by the disease, unexpected cures can rarely be attributed to any one factor: the nature of the care received, the treatment(s) delivered, specific disease or patient characteristics, or environmental or social influences. From a personal perspective, however, I have come to understand that the capacity to heal is based in part on a successful patient-doctor partnership" [27].

Dennis calls "the sweet success" of her collaboration with Dr. Neiderhuber and her primary care physician "the tipping point toward healing versus the inevitable march toward my prognosis." Yet, she sounded a wistful note in a letter to me: "It has bothered me a great deal," she wrote, "that when this patient has documented evidence to support physiologic change that falls outside the margins of accepted allopathic paradigms, no one seems to have any questions. Perhaps I am naïve ... but you would think medicine would be intensely interested in people who have done what they said couldn't be done" [28]. I could only reply to her that I felt certain the day was not far off.

References

[1] Lerner M. Choices in healing. Cambridge (UK): MIT Press; 1994. p. 841.

[2] Rosenberg SA, Fox E, Churchill WH. Spontaneous regression of hepatic metastases from gastric carcinoma. Cancer 1972;29(2):472–4.

[3] Rosenberg SA, Anderson WF, Blaese M, et al. The development of gene therapy for the treatment of cancer. Ann Surg 1993;218(4):455–64.

[4] Kissane DW, Grabsch B, Clarke DM, et al. Supportive-expressive group therapy for women with metastatic breast cancer: survival and psychosocial outcome from a randomized controlled trial. Psychooncology 2007;16(4):277–86.

[5] Spiegel D, Butler LD, Giese-Davis J, et al. Effects of supportive-expressive group therapy on survival of patients with metastatic breast cancer: a randomized prospective trial. Cancer 2007;110(5):1130–8.

[6] Allday E. Group therapy not a boost to cancer survival after all: psychological support doesn't extend life for most breast patients, says researcher. San Francisco Chronicle. July 23, 2007; p. D-1.

[7] Staren ED, Essner R, Economou JS. Overview of biological response modifiers. Semin Surg Oncol 2006;5(6):379–84, published online.

[8] Everson T, Cole W. Spontaneous regression of cancer. Philadelphia: WB Saunders Co.; 1966. p. 519–20.

[9] Coley WB. The treatment of inoperable sarcoma by bacterial toxins (the mixed toxins of streptococcus of erysipilus and the bacillus prodigiosus). Practitioner 1909;(83):589–613.

[10] Hirshberg C, Barasch MI. Remarkable Recovery. New York: Riverhead Books; 1995. p. 52–258.

[11] Niethe U. [Spontaneous healing of a malignoma?]. Klin Monatsbl Augenheilkd 1975;166(1):137–8 [in German].

[12] Foster H. Lifestyle changes and the "spontaneous" regression of cancer: an initial computer analysis. International Journal of Biosocial Medicine 1988;10(1):17–33.

[13] Hildenbrand G, Hildenbrand L. Five-year survival rates of melanoma patients treated by diet therapy after the manner of Gerson: a retrospective review. Alternative Therapies 1995; V1. The authors report that of 35 Stage III melanoma cases, 5-year survival rate was 71% compared with the 5-year survivals of the following studies: The American Cancer Society, 39%; Brisbane, 27%; and Duke University, 42%.

[14] Groopman J. Faith and healing. New York Times Book Review 2008;27:1–2.

[15] Hall HR, et al. Voluntary modulation of neutrophil adhesiveness using a cyberphysiologic strategy. Int J Neurosci 1992;63:287–97.

[16] Ogston K, Walker MB, Simpson E, et al. A controlled clinical trial of the immunological effects of relaxation training and guided imagery in women with locally advanced breast cancer. Eur J Surg Oncol 1997;(23):372.

[17] Walker LG, Walker MB, Ogston K, et al. Psychological, clinical and pathological effects of relaxation training and guided imagery during primary chemotherapy. Br J Cancer 1999;80:262–8.

[18] Forlenza MJ, Baum A. Psychosocial influences on cancer progression: alternative cellular and molecular mechanisms. Curr Opin Psychiatry 2000;13(6):639–45.

[19] Temoshok LR. Complex coping patterns and their role in adaptation and neuroimmunomodulation: theory, methodology, and research. Ann N Y Acad Sci 2000;917:446–55.

[20] Goodwin JS, et al. The effect of marital status on stage, treatment and survival of cancer patients. JAMA 1987;258(21):125–31.

[21] Goleman D. Doctors find comfort is a potent medicine. The New York Times. February 16, 1991; p. B5, B8.

[22] Kiecolt-Glaser JK, Malarkey WB, Chee M, et al. Negative behavior during marital conflict is associated with immunological down-regulation. Psychosom Med 1993;55(5):395–409.

[23] Lutgendorf SK, Sood AK, Anderson B, et al. Social support, psychological distress, and natural killer cell activity in ovarian cancer. J Clin Oncol 2005;23(28):7105–13.

[24] Cousins N. Head first: the biology of hope and the healing power of the human spirit. New York: Dutton; 1989. p. 122–6.

[25] We cite in Remarkable Recovery (p. 36–38) an unusual, religiously tinged remission attested to by leukemia pioneer Dr. Sidney Farber, but never reported in the medical literature. Hematologist Dr. Milton Sacks, who treated the case, told a *Washington Post* reporter in 1993, "The only reason this case has not been written up is that I have been afraid to." Jones T, The saint and Ann O'Neill. The Washington Post, April 3, 1994: V1–F5.

[26] Bell JW. Possible immune factors in a spontaneous regression of bronchogenic carcinoma: ten-year survival in a patient treated with minimal (1,200r) radiation alone. Am J Surg 1970;120:804–6.

[27] Niederhuber JE, private correspondence, 2007, April 10, quoted with permission.

[28] Dennis K, author correspondence, 2008,18 January, quoted with permission.

Hematol Oncol Clin N Am 22 (2008) 767–773

HEMATOLOGY/ONCOLOGY CLINICS
OF NORTH AMERICA

Practicing a Medicine of the Whole Person: An Opportunity for Healing

Rachel Naomi Remen, MD[a,b,*]

[a]Institute for the Study of Health and Illness at Commonweal, Box 316, Bolinas, CA 94924, USA
[b]Department of Family and Community Medicine, University of California, San Francisco, 500 Parnassus Avenue, MU 3E, San Francisco, CA 94143-0900, USA

"Inspire me with love for all of thy creatures, May I see in all who suffer only the fellow human being."

From the Prayer of Maimonedes

Integrative medicine has been defined in several ways. For some it is a discipline that combines such approaches to the resolution of disease as acupuncture and homeopathy, meditation, and imagery with more familiar and accepted health practices, such as surgery, pediatrics, and oncology. For others it is about cultivating awareness and sensitivity beyond symptoms to the mental, emotional, and spiritual needs of the patient. Integrative medicine, however, is more than the weaving together of techniques, or understanding the intimate interaction of the mental, emotional, and spiritual dimensions of human experience. Integrative medicine is about rethinking the task of medicine and the infrastructure of relationships and beliefs that have limited its power to serve all people.

For the past 100 years medicine has focused on the expertise and techniques that can affect the cure of the body. But, in oncology, cure is not always possible. In the absence of cure we are challenged to care for people living with problems they might have died of only a short time ago. Our training has not prepared us to do this and so it is not surprising that many chronically ill patients believe that contemporary medicine has little to offer them except symptom management.

Integrative oncology is not only about cancer. It is also about the people who have cancer and those that love them, and the transformative impact of this disease on their lives. Integrative oncology is a medicine of the whole person. It is about recognizing that personal wholeness and physical limitation often coexist and moving the focus of care beyond the cure of the body to the healing of the whole person. It is about inviting our patients into our examining rooms

*ISHI/Commonweal, Box 316, Bolinas, CA 94924. *E-mail address:* drrachel@commonweal.org

0889-8588/08/$ – see front matter
doi:10.1016/j.hoc.2008.04.001

hemonc.theclinics.com

as whole people and meeting them there as whole people. It is about recognizing that as whole people, we bring a far greater capacity to meet with the challenge of disease than we have been trained to recognize.

Disease is often an agent of personal transformation. In the presence of physical illness people can grow as persons in their capacity to love, their compassion, their sensitivity and understanding, their courage and wisdom. Because of this capacity for growth it often is possible for chronically ill people to live beyond the limitations of their disease.

Some time ago one of my patients spontaneously discovered this for himself in the form of a dream. David was 16 when he was diagnosed with juvenile diabetes. Almost immediately his disease became an absolute authority in his life, telling him what to eat, how much to exercise, requiring him to stop and test himself over and over in the course of a single day. David was an adolescent and his response to this was rage. He flung himself against the limitations of his disease like an animal trapped in a cage. He refused to hold to a diet, he skipped doses of insulin, played ball, and partied with his friends with no consideration of his diabetes. Not surprisingly, he appeared in the emergency room in coma or shock almost every month. Fearing for his life his parents insisted he enter therapy. He did not want to do this, but he came.

For the first 6 months we met weekly. Every week, he would silently sit in my office without meeting my eyes for a full hour. I sat in silence as well, secretly admiring his passion and his determination to live a full life. Then one week, after 15 minutes of his usual silence, he looked up and offered to share a dream he had the previous night. He had dreamt that he was sitting alone in an empty room opposite a small stone statue of the Buddha. When I asked him how he felt, he described a feeling of kinship with the statue because the statue depicted the Buddha as a young man, not much older then himself.

"Is there a word that describes the statue?" I asked. He paused to consider. "Peaceful," he said and told me that sitting opposite it caused him to feel peaceful too. In his dream, he sat and enjoyed this unfamiliar sense of peace for some time, and then without warning, a knife was thrown from somewhere behind him. It buried itself deep in the heart of the Buddha.

David was horrified and flooded with painful feelings. Despite this he could not look away and as he watched, it seemed to him that the Buddha was getting larger. It was so slow that at first he was not sure that it was really happening, but so it was. And somehow, in the way of dreams, he knew without doubt that this growth was the Buddha's response to the knife. The peaceful expression on the Buddha's face never changed and neither did the knife. Gradually it became a tiny black dot on the breast of this enormous smiling Buddha. Watching this David felt something release him and found he could breathe deeply for the first time in a long time. When he awoke he found tears in his eyes.

David was intrigued by the dream and at first did not recognize its meaning. As we spoke he realized that the feelings of despair and shock and betrayal he had felt when the knife plunged into the heart of the Buddha were the same feelings he had experienced in his doctor's office when he had learned that he had diabetes and that it was incurable. But his reaction to his diagnosis had been far different than the Buddha's reaction to the knife.

David saw this dream as the opening of a door. When he received his diagnosis he had felt stopped, as if there was no way for him to move forward. It had seemed to him that the only way that he might recover a life would be to rebel against this disease with all of his strength. But the dream had shown him something different. It suggested over time he might grow in such a way that his disease could become a smaller and smaller part of the sum total of his life; that perhaps he might be able to live a good life even if it was not going to be an easy life or a long life. Integrative medicine has the potential of opening a door of hope for oncology patients as well.

The normalization of physiology, the longtime goal of medicine, may be only a part of our potential to make a difference in the lives of others. Integrative medicine is about serving all people, not only those we can cure. It goes far beyond the cure of the body to the recognition of the potential for growth in everyone and involves a commitment on the part of health professionals to support that growth by all means possible. Integrative medicine is about nothing less than reclaiming healing as the primary goal of care.

There is a real difference between healing and curing. The goal of cure is optimal physical function. The goal of healing is the capacity to live a full and meaningful life, an end point often within reach even in the absence of cure. In the presence of chronic illness it is not unusual for people to discover a capacity to live more richly, fully, and passionately than ever before. This evolution of the individual is a part of the human response to disease and may be a function of that mysterious human dimension, the will to live.

The will to live awakens in response to the challenge of disease. Sometimes, it takes the form of physiologic resolution, but more often it is present in far subtler forms, such as a shift in values and priorities, which allows a far greater range of response to life.

Another of my patients, a successful executive, told me that his life before cancer was an unending pursuit of "the cookie." Happiness was "having the cookie." If you had the cookie, things were good. If you did not have the cookie, life was not worth a damn. Some times the cookie was money, sometimes power, sometimes sex. Sometimes, it was the new car, the biggest contract, and the most prestigious address. It was never enough. A year and a half after his diagnosis of prostate cancer he sits shaking his head ruefully. "The cookie never made me happy for long," he tells me. "The minute I had it, I began to worry about someone taking it away from me. Often I never got a chance to eat it because I was so busy just trying not to lose it."

My patient laughed and said that cancer has changed him. For the first time he is truly happy. No matter if his business is doing well or not, no matter if he wins or if he loses at golf. "Two years ago, cancer asked me 'OK, Sol, what is important? What is really important?' Well, life is important. Life. Life any way you can have it. Life with the cookie, life without the cookie. Happiness does not have anything to do with the cookie; it has to do with being alive.

Before, who made the time?" He pauses thoughtfully. "Damn, I guess life IS the cookie."

Cancer can evoke personal growth in the families around our patients as well. In the presence of this disease, people step past lifelong limitations and may come to know themselves and recognize their capacities for the first time.

From the moment he was diagnosed with non-Hodgkin's lymphoma Richard was concerned about his wife Alice. He described her as painfully shy and almost housebound. He could not imagine how she would be able to deal with the possibility of his death and should he die how she could manage alone with their children and the very successful business he had developed.

When I first met Alice she was so timid that she was unable to look directly at me. I could not imagine how she might cope either. Yet, as Richard lost ground and disappointment after disappointment led to his premature death, she underwent a remarkable change. It was she who supported him in taking necessary risks; she who researched experimental treatments and reached out to experts around the country; she who took over more and more of his business, learning as she went; she who supported and comforted their children. Her courage, both in her personal and her business life, was as awesome as it was unexpected. By the time he died she was running the business and afterward continued to make a success of it alone.

A few years after he died, I met her at a party. She was simply not the woman who had come to my office only 3 years before. I commented on the remarkable strength she had shown in dealing with her husband's illness and death and making a life for herself and her family. Had she known that she would be able to do this?

"Well, no," she said. She had always been painfully shy from the time she was a small girl. Everyone knew this so no one had ever challenged her and she had never challenged herself. Yet, her courage and her ability to take risks had come very naturally to her. She had been surprised at first, but then she had decided that her bravery was a result of her shyness. She smiled. "I was so shy that it took courage for me to say 'hello' to someone, it took courage to go to the supermarket and to the cleaners, it felt like a risk every time I answered the telephone. It took a lot of courage just to live, to do the things that other people do without thinking every day. I guess over the years my courage just grew from being used all the time like that. And when the time came that Richard needed me so badly, when I could no longer help him and be shy, why I guess I was ready."

Healing is about engaging the will to live in others, something that we do with our humanity and not with our expertise. We can profoundly affect the personal wholeness in others in very simple ways. We heal most often with our listening and our presence. When we listen to others without judgment, simply to know what is true for them at this time in their lives, we may enable them to hear their personal truth, and recognize their strength often for the first time. When we are present as vulnerable and whole people, we may enable others to accept their present vulnerability without diminishing their strength.

A physician who herself has a significant chronic illness told me of asking a newly diagnosed patient how he felt about having cancer. "Ashamed," he replied. Months later this same patient told her that he no longer felt this way. When she asked what had made the difference, the patient had replied, "When I first met you I had thought you were whole and I was broken. Now that I know you too have a story, I no longer feel ashamed of mine. I know I am not singled out or broken or alone."

In the presence of a whole person no one need feel ashamed of their vulnerability or alone with their pain. Oftentimes the will to live is weakened more by isolation than by disease.

Most of us are not aware of the power of our personal humanity to strengthen others to meet with the altered circumstances of their lives. Our training suggests that our expertise is all we have to offer patients. But healing is not a relationship between an expert and a problem. It is the outcome of meeting as two whole people who recognize the potential in their relationship to exceed the limitations of both science and disease. Our humanity includes both our strengths and our vulnerabilies. In the archetype of the wounded healer, Jung suggests that wounded people can best be healed by other wounded people. It is the wisdom gained from one's own wounds and experiences of suffering that make us able to trust the process of healing even in the darkest of times, not as a theory but as a personal experience. Our own wounds teach us compassion for the wounds of others and allow us to recognize the strengths that may develop in times of weakness and despair. After years of working with chronically ill people, I have found that my expertise has turned out to be less important to long range outcomes than becoming genuinely present and remembering and trusting the hidden capacity for growth in myself and everyone else.

The healing relationship is mutual. Over time curing is often draining but healing is renewing. When we cure people, we grow in skill, but our healing relationships develop our humanity and deepen our appreciation of the meaning of our work.

Much in medical training prevents us from seeing the meaning in the work that we do daily. We are trained to objectivity, to a certain emotional distance. We take refuge in the cognitive, the dimension of fact and analysis, and are uncomfortable with things that are not measurable and replicable.

Yet, the meaning of our work lies in its human connections. Finding meaning requires us to bring more of ourselves to our work than is often our custom. This is no easy transformation, because many of us are products of a training that actively discouraged this sort of presence. I emerged from my training with the firm view that a genuine human connection with my patients was unprofessional. But the courage to connect in this way may be the key to finding the deepest meaning and satisfaction in our work. It is not surprising that most of us live far more meaningful lives than we know.

The world of meaning is not made up of facts; the world of meaning is made up of stories. Stories of heroism, courage, devotion, and strength surround us daily, the sort of stories that can be appreciated only by a fellow human being. No two people with the same disease have the same story. Finding the meaning of our work does not require us to do anything differently. It may simply require us to see familiar things in new ways.

There is a deep river of meaning that runs through our daily work. Sometimes the simplest of techniques can give us new eyes and remind us of the meaning that lies just below the surface of our work. Hundreds of physicians have found a greater meaning in their work through a commitment to keep a brief and simple journal. All that is required is spending 10 minutes at the end of each day reviewing the events of the day three times, each time asking yourself a different question. The first time, ask the question "What surprised me today?" The second time, ask "What touched my heart today?" The third time, ask "What inspired me today?" As soon as you find the first thing that answers your question, you stop your review and write it down. Then you go back to the start of your day and begin your review again, asking yourself the next question.

This simple technique saved Richard's career. A highly successful oncologic surgeon, he had become so depressed that he felt unable to go on. "I drag myself out of bed each morning," he told me. "I have to get out of this game." When I suggested he keep this journal he was highly dubious but agreed to try. A week after our conversation he called to ask me if there was some trick to this. "Why, what do you mean, Richard?" I asked.

Reluctantly, he reported that day after day he had gotten the same answer to all three questions "Nothing, nothing, and nothing." "How can I be so busy and lead such a boring life?" he demanded. "Are you looking at the events of your day as if you are a doctor?" I asked. "Of course," he snapped. I laughed. "Well try looking as if you are a novelist or a poet. Look for the stories," I told him. The telephone went silent. "I'll try," he said.

Surprisingly, I did not hear from Richard again for a number of weeks, and then he called to thank me. His voice, usually flat, had changed. "How are things?" I asked. "The same but different" he replied.

He told me then of the transformation he had experienced in his work. It had taken a while, but eventually he began to find answers to all three questions. At first, the only thing that surprised him was that a tumor had shrunk on x-ray or chemotherapy had unexpectedly worked. But then, he had begun to notice other things. The warmth that lit up a patient's face when he walked into the examining room, the way a little girl was dressed as if she was gift wrapped in her go-to-church best whenever she was brought to his office, the bond between an 83-year-old patient and his 80-year-old wife who held each others arthritic hands throughout their visit. "Its all about love," he told me, "people's love for each other and their love for me whether I can cure them or not. And its about my love for them too. I had not known. I had thought it was all about cancer."

Perhaps taking an integrative approach to health care does more than introduce healing into our relationships. It allows us to reclaim our lineage and furthers the healing of medicine itself. Many years ago in a classics course I read the description of the Temples of Aescalapius, the father of medicine, offered in the writings of Cicero. I was surprised to discover that in the central courtyard of this most ancient of medical centers stood a statue of Venus, the goddess of love. As a young doctor this had puzzled me, but now after 46 years of doctoring the wisdom in it seems clear and unchanged by the passage of time. For all of its scientific power, medicine is not a work of science. Medicine is a work of service, and serving the life in others is a special kind of love.

HEMATOLOGY/ONCOLOGY CLINICS
OF NORTH AMERICA

INDEX

Note: Page numbers of article titles are in **boldface** type.

0889-8588/08/$ – see front matter
doi:10.1016/S0889-8588(08)00092-0